MAXIMAL MYOCARDIAL PERFUSION AS A MEASURE OF THE FUNCTIONAL SIGNIFICANCE OF CORONARY ARTERY DISEASE

Developments in Cardiovascular Medicine

VOLUME 127

The titles published in this series are listed at the end of this volume.

Maximal Myocardial Perfusion as a Measure of the Functional Significance of Coronary Artery Disease

From a Pathoanatomic to a Pathophysiologic Interpretation of the Coronary Arteriogram

by

NICO H.J. PIJLS
Department of Cardiology, University Hospital Nijmegen,
Nijmegen, The Netherlands

Forewords by K. Lance Gould and Steven E. Nissen

KLUWER ACADEMIC PUBLISHERS
DORDRECHT / BOSTON / LONDON

Library of Congress Cataloging-in-Publication Data

Pijls, Nico H. J., 1952-
    Maximal myocardial perfusion as a measure of the fuctional
significance of coronary artery disease : from a pathoanatomic to a
pathophysiological interpretation of the coronary arteriogram / by
Nico H.J. Pijls ; foreword by K. Lance Gould and Steven E. Nissen.
    p. cm. -- (Developments in cardovascular medicine ; v. 127)
    Includes index.
    ISBN 0-7923-1430-1 (hb : alk. paper)
    1. Coronary heart disease. 2. Coronary circulation--Measurement.
3. Angiocardiography.   I. Title.   II. Series.
    [DNLM: 1. Blood Flow Velocity. 2. Blood Volume Determination-
-methods. 3. Coronary Disease--diagnosis. 4. Coronary Disease-
-physiopathology. 5. Heart--radionuclide imaging. 6. Densitometry,
X-Ray.   W1 DE997VME v. 127 / WG 300 P63m]
RC685.C6P54 1991
616.1'23--dc20
DNLM/DLC
for Library of Congress   91-20891

ISBN 0-7923-1430-1

Published by Kluwer Academic Publishers,
P.O. Box 17, 3300 AA Dordrecht, The Netherlands.

Kluwer Academic Publishers incorporates
the publishing programmes of
D. Reidel, Martinus Nijhoff, Dr W. Junk and MTP Press.

Sold and distributed in the U.S.A. and Canada
by Kluwer Academic Publishers,
101 Philip Drive, Norwell, MA 02061, U.S.A.

In all other countries, sold and distributed
by Kluwer Academic Publishers Group
P.O. Box 322, 3300 AH Dordrecht, The Netherlands.

Printed on acid-free paper

Dedicated to
All who taught me

Contents

Forewords   **xi**

List of abbreviations   **xv**

1 Introduction   **1**
  1.1   The limited value of classical coronary arteriography to predict
       the physiologic significance of coronary artery stenoses.   1
  1.2   Coronary flow reserve   4
  1.3   Maximal coronary and myocardial blood flow   5

2 Methods of Measuring Myocardial Blood Flow   **13**
  2.1   Laboratory methods   13
      2.1.1   Timed venous collection   13
      2.1.2   Electromagnetic flow measurement   14
      2.1.3   Epicardial ultrasonic flow velocity measurement   14
      2.1.4   Microspheres   16
  2.2   Clinical methods   18
      2.2.1   Coronary sinus thermodilution   19
      2.2.2   Gas clearance methods   19
      2.2.3   The Doppler catheter   20
      2.2.4   Videodensitometry   21
      2.2.5   Positron emission tomography   21
      2.2.6   Other methods   22

**3 Application of Indicator Dilution Theory in the Investigation
of the Cardiovascular System**   **27**
  3.1   History   27
  3.2   The two approaches in indicator dilution theory   28
      3.2.1   Measurement of Flow   29
      3.2.2   Measurement of Volume   31
      3.2.3   Calculation of Mean Transit Time   32
  3.3   Videodensitometry and digital arteriography for flow assessment
       in the coronary circulation   33

4 Problems and Limitations in the Application of Videodensitometry to Assess Coronary Blood Flow and Myocardial Perfusion   **39**

4.1   Influence of the contrast agent on flow   40

4.2   Changes in vascular volume   42

4.3   Contrast density vs contrast concentration   43

4.4   Difficulties in determination of mean transit time due to motion and insufficient image quality   45

4.5   Prerequisites for myocardial flow assessment by videodensitometry, according to the physiology of indicator dilution theory   .   47

5 A Model Study to Validate Calculation of Myocardial Blood Flow by Videodensitometry   **53**

5.1   Introduction   53

5.2   Materials and methods   55

    5.2.1   Flow model   55

    5.2.2   Image acquisition and processing   55

    5.2.3   Absorption characteristics   57

    5.2.4   Processing of time-density curves   57

    5.2.5   Relation between flow and time parameters   58

5.3   Results   59

    5.3.1   Applicability of Lambert-Beer's law   59

    5.3.2   Fitting of the curves   59

    5.3.3   Assessment of relative flow   59

    5.3.4   Assessment of absolute flow   61

5.4   Discussion   62

5.5   Conclusions   66

6 Mean Transit Time for the Assessment of Myocardial Perfusion by Videodensitometry   **71**

6.1   Introduction   71

6.2   Methods   73

    6.2.1   Animal instrumentation and experimental protocol . . .   73

    6.2.2   Achievement of constant vascular volume and different flow levels   74

    6.2.3   Image acquisition and image processing   75

    6.2.4   Processing of regions of interest and time-density curves   76

    6.2.5   Data processing and statistical analysis   80

6.3   Results   81

    6.3.1   Hemodynamic observations and verification of the animal model   81

    6.3.2   Quality of image acquisition and time-density curves . .   82

    6.3.3   Relation between inverse mean transit time and flow . .   86

6.3.4 Relation between $1/T_{app}^{(1)}$, $1/T_{app}^{(2)}$, $1/T_{app}^{(3)}$, D_{max} , $D_{max}/T_{app}^{(1)}$, $D_{max}/T_{app}^{(2)}$, $D_{max}/T_{app}^{(3)}$, $1/T_{max}$ and flow ... 86

6.4 Discussion 91

6.5 Clinical implications and limitations 95

7 The Concept of Maximal Flow Ratio for Immediate Evaluation of PTCA Result ... **101**

7.1 Introduction 101

7.2 Methods 102

    7.2.1 Patient population and study design 102

    7.2.2 Image acquisition and processing 103

    7.2.3 Processing of the regions of interest and time-density curves. 104

    7.2.4 Data processing and statistical analysis 105

7.3 Results 108

    7.3.1 Clinical and hemodynamic data 108

    7.3.2 Quality and reproducibility of image acquisition and time-density curves 109

    7.3.3 Relation between MFR and exercise tests results 113

    7.3.4 Comparison of T_{mn} belonging to apparently normal arteries and to stenotic arteries before and after successful PTCA 117

7.4 Discussion 117

7.5 Limitations 120

8 Reproducibility of Mean Transit Time for Maximal Myocardial Flow Assessment ... **129**

8.1 Introduction 129

8.2 Methods 130

    8.2.1 Study protocol and image acquisition 130

    8.2.2 Image processing and processing of TDCs 131

    8.2.3 Data processing and statistical analysis 132

8.3 Results 134

8.4 Discussion 137

9 General Discussion ... **141**

9.1 Discussion 141

9.2 Conclusions 143

9.3 Limitations 143

9.4 Spin-off and Present Applications 145

A Is Nonionic Isotonic Iohexol the Contrast Agent of Choice for Quantitative Myocardial Videodensitometry? ... **151**

A.1 Introduction 151

A.2 Methods 153
     A.2.1 Animal preparation and instrumentation 153
     A.2.2 Contrast injections 154
     A.2.3 Hemodynamic recordings 154
     A.2.4 Statistical analysis 155
A.3 Results 155
     A.3.1 Baseline values and reactions to verapamil 155
     A.3.2 Effect of contrast injections on coronary blood flow . . . 156
     A.3.3 Effect of contrast injections on left ventricular
            $(dP/dt)_{max}$, left ventricular systolic pressure, and heart
            rate 157
     A.3.4 Reaction to 20 seconds coronary artery occlusion 159
     A.3.5 Relation between change in coronary blood flow and change
            in left ventricular $(dP/dt)_{max}$ 161
A.4 Discussion 161
A.5 Conclusion 164

B Fitting Procedures for Time-Density Curves   167

Summary   173

Index   181

Foreword

Coronary flow reserve is a functional measure of stenosis severity reflecting the integrated effects of its geometry including percent stenosis, absolute lumen area, length and shape. Its clinical application has been primarily qualitative in non-invasive, perfusion imaging.

Measurement of coronary flow reserve during routine coronary arteriography has been an elusive goal. Transit time and indicator dilution techniques for assessing coronary flow reserve at cardiac catheterization are associated with marked variability compared to microspheres or flow meters, thereby making their use questionable in comparison to the precision of good quantitative arteriography. Coronary flow reserve measured by special Doppler catheters as an adjunct to coronary arteriography shows in man the value of this integrated functional measure of stenosis severity and the limitations of percent diameter narrowing as a measure of its physiologic significance. However, Doppler catheters require additional instrumentation that is not yet an integral part of coronary arteriography and provide measures of absolute coronary flow reserve only.

Relative maximum flow or relative flow reserve has been demonstrated to be an important independent, complimentary descriptor of stenosis severity independent of fluctuating hemodynamic conditions. The method developed for DSA by Nico Pijls, described in this book is the first approach for assessing relative coronary flow reserve as a part of routine coronary arteriography by DSA. The theory and basic concepts are well developed, experimental validation thorough and clinical applications timely.

Perhaps most importantly this superb monograph illustrates the scientific imagination and meticulous methodology that builds on existing knowledge and advances our understanding of the field. It makes a substantial contribution and should be in the library of every cardiologist interested in coronary pathophysiology.

K. Lance Gould, M.D.
Professor of Medicine
University of Texas Medical School at Houston

Foreword

Although arteriography is widely used to assess the severity of coronary artery disease (CAD), radiographic evaluation of coronary anatomy has many limitations. Angiography records only a silhouette of the vessel lumen, and can misrepresent the extent of complex coronary narrowings. Studies have shown large observer variability in the interpretation of angiograms and important discrepancies with postmortem histology. The severity of lesions is expressed as percent stenosis, but there is often no "normal segment" with which to compare a focal narrowing and percent stenosis may therefore underestimate disease severity. Accordingly, studies have documented a poor correlation between percent stenosis and the physiological consequences of lesions.

The limitations of stenosis sizing by angiography have led several investigators to examine videodensitometry as a means to assess the physiology of coronary lesions. Contrast density-time curves from digital angiography (DSA) are used to determine coronary flow reserve (CFR), defined as the ratio of coronary blood flow (CBF) following pharmacologic vasodilation divided by CBF under basal conditions. Multiple alternative approaches for assessment of CFR have been introduced, but none have achieved widespread acceptance.

Several problems have impeded optimal application of DSA to assessment of CFR. The physiologic effects of contrast injection complicate DSA techniques. Epicardial passage of contrast first reduces CBF, then induces an intense hyperemic response. Most DSA methods to evaluate flow have employed an approach based upon the transit-time of a contrast bolus. Several investigators have measured a phenomenon termed "myocardial contrast appearance- time" (MCAT), defined as the time interval between onset of contrast injection and the time at which density in a myocardial region of interest (ROI) reaches a certain percent of maximum. However, vasodilation of the coronary resistance bed during contrast passage increases the apparent volume of distribution of contrast media, an important confounding variable. More importantly, MCAT does not reflect any well established physiologic principles of flow.

Additional problems have hindered clinical application of DSA methods for CFR determination. All of the previous approaches calculate CFR defined as the ratio of hyperemic to basal flow. Unfortunately, a reduced CFR can be produced by two phenomena: reduction in hyperemic flow by an epicardial stenosis or increased basal flow produced by factors unrelated to the lesion. Many factors including left ventricular hypertrophy, tachycardia or valvular heart disease can reduce CFR measurements in clinical decision-making.

In this book, Pijls and colleagues have systematically investigated a new and exciting approach to CBF analysis. They avoid measuring CFR as a descriptor of the functional significance of coronary lesions. Instead they measure mean myocardial transit-time during continuous maximal coronary vasodilation induced by infusion of dipyridamole or papaverine. Instead of yielding measurements of CFR, their method yields a value representative of the maximal possible flow achievable for the analyzed vascular bed. The mean transit-time approach is well founded in physiologic principles and Pijls has carefully considered each of the potential confounding variables.

The clinical implications of the studies by Pijls et al are significant. The method can provide a measurement of maximal possible flow for a given stenosis both prior to and following balloon angioplasty. In this application, the extent of functional improvement can be assessed immediately following angioplasty and used to predict the long-term success of interventional procedures. Accordingly, this new approach adds an important tool to the diagnostic armamentarium. Coronary surgery and balloon angioplasty are among the most common and costly therapeutic procedures in current practice. Clinical decision-making regarding interventional procedures is optimal only when both anatomic and functional data are available. The mean transit-time approach pioneered by Pijls et al appears to offer considerable value and will likely undergo further development and application in coming years.

Steven E. Nissen
Associate professor of Medicine
University of Kentucky Medical Center

List of abbreviations

AoP	: aortic pressure
BCM	: background region of interest to the myocardium,
	: supplied by the left circumflex artery
BLM	: background region of interest to the myocardium,
	: supplied by the left anterior descending artery
CFR	: coronary flow reserve
CM	: region of interest over the myocardium, supplied
	: by the left circumflex artery
D_{max}	: maximal contrast density
DSA	: digital subtraction angiography
EM	: electromagnetic
E_r	: relative error
ET	: exercise test
F	: flow
f_d	: Doppler shift
LAD	: left anterior descending artery
LCA	: left coronary artery
LAO	: left anterior oblique
LM	: region of interest over the myocardium, supplied
	: by the left anterior descending artery
LCx	: left circumflex artery
LV dP/dt	: first derivative of the left ventricular pressure
LV dP/dt$_{max}$	: maximal positive LV dp/dt
LVP	: left ventricular pressure
M	: amount of injected indicator
MFR	: maximal flow ratio
MFR_c	: maximal flow ratio after correction for
	: pressure changes
NYHA	: New York Heart Association

O-140	: the contrast agent Iohexol-140
O-350	: the contrast agent Iohexol-350
P	: pressure
P_a	: arterial pressure
PET	: positron emission tomography
PTCA	: percutaneous transluminal coronary angioplasty
RAO	: right anterior oblique
RCA	: right coronary artery
ROI	: region of interest
T_{app}	: appearance time of contrast agent
TDC	: time density curve
T_{max}	: time of maximal concentration of contrast agent
T_{mn}	: mean transit time of contrast agent between
	: an injection site and a measuring site
U-370	: the contrast agent diatrizoate-370
V	: volume of the vascular bed between an injection
	: site of an indicator and a measuring site.

Chapter 1

Introduction

1.1 The limited value of classical coronary arteriography to predict the physiologic significance of coronary artery stenoses.

Since its development in the early 1960s, coronary arteriography has been of great importance in the diagnosis and management of patients with ischemic heart disease [1, 2, 3]. Also for the next decade, it can be expected that, once the functional significance of a stenosis has been proved, anatomic data obtained at arteriography will remain necessary as a map for the cardiac surgeon or the interventional cardiologist to be informed about the correct sites where bypasses have to be placed or the balloon has to be inflated.

Despite this acknowledged pivotal role of coronary arteriography to locate a stenosis, the functional significance of an arteriographic lesion cannot be settled from the arteriogram alone [3, 4]. The primary method for validating the arteriographic interpretation of coronary lesions has been to compare the angiographic data with postmortem anatomic data [5, 6, 7]. In these studies, severe underestimation as well as overestimation was encountered [5, 6, 7, 8, 9, 10]. Furthermore, a large intraobserver and interobserver variability has been documented in many studies [11, 12, 13]. More recently, a number of well documented studies have confirmed a poor correlation between anatomic estimation of coronary narrowings and physiologic measures of coronary function [14, 15]. It is generally agreed that the limitations of arteriography are most troublesome for stenoses of 50-90% diameter narrowing, unfortunately being the range of most interest [3]. *At the present time, there remains*

1

little doubt that evaluation of coronary obstructions by quantitation of anatomic luminal narrowing represents a fundamentally flawed approach [16].

A number of explanations have been considered for the discrepancy between anatomic severity and the physiologic significance of a coronary stenosis. Some of these can be attributed to the inherent shortcomings of regular cineangiographic methods to reconstruct 3-dimensional structures from scalar planes. Inadequate focus size, orientation of vessels to X-ray direction, stenoses in curved segments of the arterial tree, and asymmetrical narrowing (figure 1.1A) all contribute to possible mistakes in stenosis assessment [17]. Due to the curvilinear relation between diameter and resistance, the effective resistance of the lesion can vary markedly with only small - even invisible - changes in degree of narrowing, especially in the range of 70-99% stenoses. Overestimation of stenosis severity may also occur because of inadequate filling of the vessel with contrast, abnormalities in coronary runoff, or concomitant coronary artery spasm.

Furthermore, percent stenosis is determined by comparing diameter in the stenotic segment to an adjacent "normal" segment. Pathologic studies, however, indicate that coronary artery disease is often diffuse with no normal segment for comparison [8, 9]. This phenomenon can lead to considerable underestimation of percent luminal narrowing [7, 10] (figure 1.1C). Although minimal coronary artery diameter has been proposed as a better prediction of the functional significance of lesions, this measure is considerably limited by the excentric, often slitlike appearance of the stenoses and by the large variability in coronary artery diameter in normal subjects [7, 9, 18].

The next point is, that it will be clear from fluid dynamics that, given a particular degree and diameter of stenosis, transstenotic pressure drop and resistance to flow can vary enormously, dependent on shape and excentricity of the lesion [19, 20] (figure 1.1B).

At last, it is important to recognize that myocardial perfusion is dependent on many other factors besides proximal coronary stenosis, such as aortic pressure, the vasodilatory capabilities of the distal myocardial vascular bed, collateral blood flow, and venous pressure. In this perspective the coronary stenosis represents but one component of a circuit in which flow depends on the function of the total system [21, 22]. Especially in the presence of a severe stenosis, where most part of the vasodilatory reserve has already been consumed, small changes in either

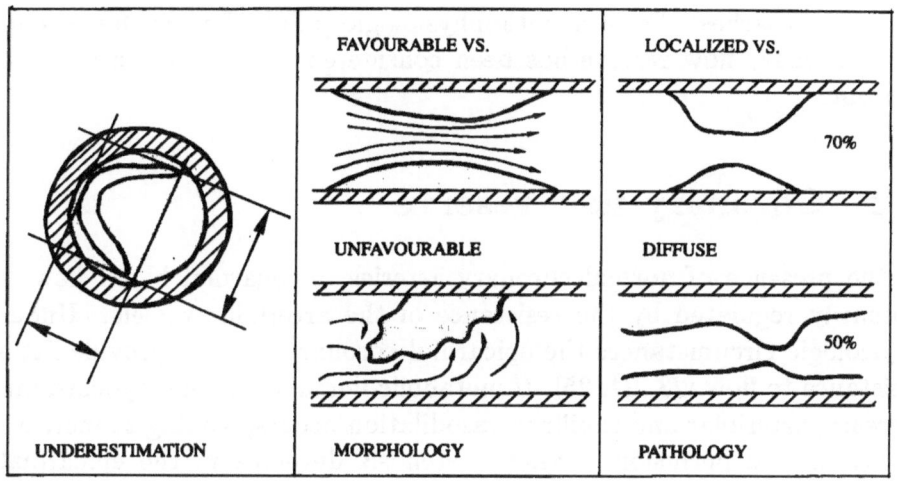

Figure 1.1: *Some explanations why the functional significance of an arterio-graphic lesion often cannot be settled from the classical coronary arteriogram alone. 1A: The morphology of the lesion resembles a semilunar slit, resulting in underestimation in every scalar plane. 1B: Pressure drop due to shear stress and flow separation is much higher if the lesion is excentric and of irregular shape, as is often the case. 1C: In the presence of diffuse disease, percentual narrowing will underestimate the significance of the lesion [19].*

arterial or venous pressure can have a large influence on flow [3].

In figure 1.2 an example is shown how classical arteriography completely fails in understanding changes in the physiologic significance of a severe coronary artery lesion. As will be shown in chapter 7, this kind of paradoxes as well as many other situations which cannot be understood from an anatomic point of view, can be solved by determining blood flow.

It may be clear now that standard anatomic methods have essential limitations in assessing the functional significance of coronary lesions. Newer, computer assisted quantitative coronary angiographic methods have diminished interobserver and intraobserver variability, but not solved this fundamental discrepancy between anatomy and physiology. To overcome these problems, many investigators have tried to obtain direct information about coronary and myocardial blood flow. A number of parameters to reflect flow have been introduced, using different approaches. From a pathophysiologic point of view, for a long time coronary flow reserve has been considered as the most attractive concept.

1.2   Coronary flow reserve

In the presence of normal coronary arteries, myocardial blood flow is primarily regulated by the resistance of the arteriolar vessels. Under physiologic circumstances the epicardial coronary arteries provide little resistance to flow [23, 24, 25]. If metabolic demands of the myocardium increase, arteriolar and capillary vasodilation occurs, leading to increase in myocardial perfusion. When a stenosis develops in the epicardial vessels, this will also lead to compensatory vasodilation distal to the stenosis and maintenance of normal resting flow to the myocardium [26].

The concept of coronary flow reserve (CFR) as a functional measure of stenosis severity was initially proposed by Gould et al in 1974 and defined as coronary blood flow after a maximal hyperemic stimulus divided by resting flow [23]. In animal studies, it could be verified that CFR under standardized hemodynamic conditions equals 500-600%, begins to decrease if stenosis severity is about 50% and continues to decrease with further increase in stenosis until approximately 90% where no reserve is present anymore [22, 26]. In the animal laboratory, CFR has been a useful concept which has provided considerable insight into a number of aspects of the coronary circulation.

In the clinical practice, however, it has become more and more obvious that the concept of CFR, despite of its theoretical correctness, has many limitations and at present its poor clinical usefulness has been largely recognized. Because CFR is defined as a ratio, diminished CFR can either mean decreased maximal flow, increased resting flow, or a combination of both. Because all methods, except PET, proposed for CFR determination in conscious man, require invasive manipulations, real resting conditions can hardly been obtained (cf. chapter 2). Contrast injection as well as introduction of Doppler catheters into coronary vessels, interfere seriously with resting flow [27, 28, 29, 30, 31, 32]. Moreover, many physiologic and pathologic conditions such as previous myocardial infarction, left ventricular hypertrophy, increased heart rate,

Figure 1.2: *(next two pages) On the left page, the coronary arteriogram and ECG are shown of a 70-year-old male, admitted with instable angina pectoris. The ECG was made within minutes before the coronary arteriogram. An apparently severe stenosis can be observed in the proximal part of the left anterior descending artery. Three days later (right page), this patient was able to perform a completely normal exercise test, without any complaints or any ECG abnormalities. The ECG at exercise (90 W; 5 min) is presented. At repeated coronary arteriography, performed immediately after the exercise test, anatomic stenosis severity seemed to be the same as before. No visible collateral circulation was present. Although the physiologic significance of this stenosis largely changed, no anatomic changes could be observed.*

and valvular disease result in an increase in resting flow and therefore in diminished CFR while vascular function can be completely normal in some of these situations [4]. Arterial hypertension influences resting flow and maximal flow. In the case of PTCA, where immediate evaluation of the result of the intervention is mandatory, the apparently resting flow is probably elevated because of long-lasting hyperemia, which can explain why CFR after PTCA does not return to normal immediately [33, 34, 35].

The main reason why coronary flow reserve has failed to become a useful concept in clinical practice, is the fundamental problem that all methods used so far to calculate this entity outside the research laboratory, significantly affect resting flow.

1.3 Maximal coronary and myocardial blood flow

One of the basic ideas in this book is that it is not resting flow or coronary flow reserve which determines the functional status of the coronary circulation, but merely the maximal flow achievable for a given part of the myocardium. The background for this idea is the simple fact that most patients with angina pectoris do not complain because of inadequate resting flow, but are limited by insufficient maximal flow through the myocardium, due to a stenosis in one of the supplying arteries. Moreover, in deciding about the success (or failure) of an intervention, it is important to know how much maximally achievable flow has increased. Therefore, maximal flow is a clinically important parameter which gives

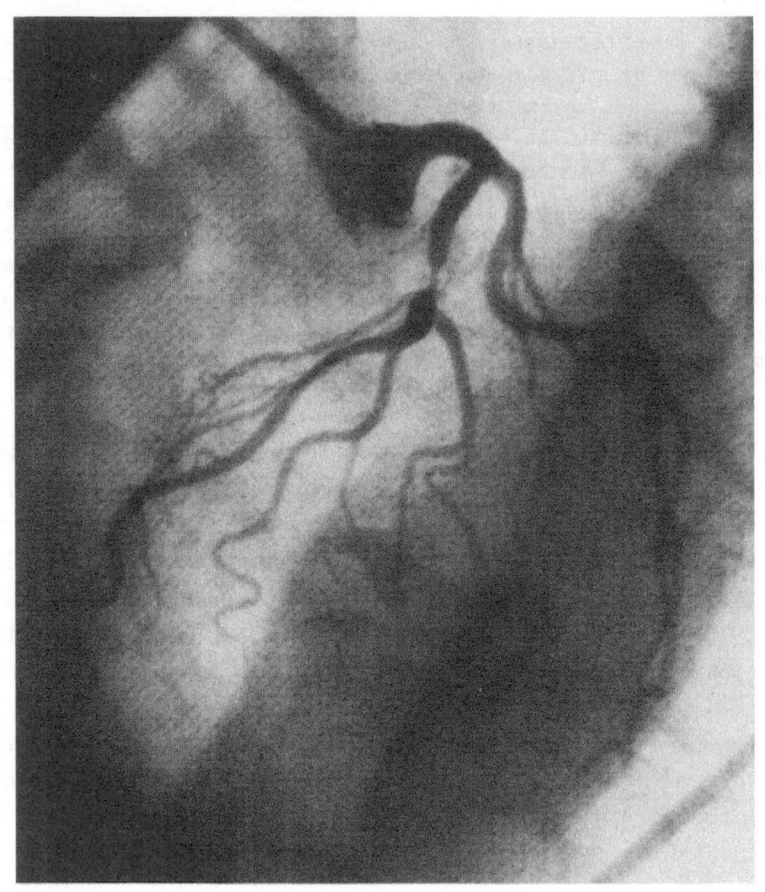

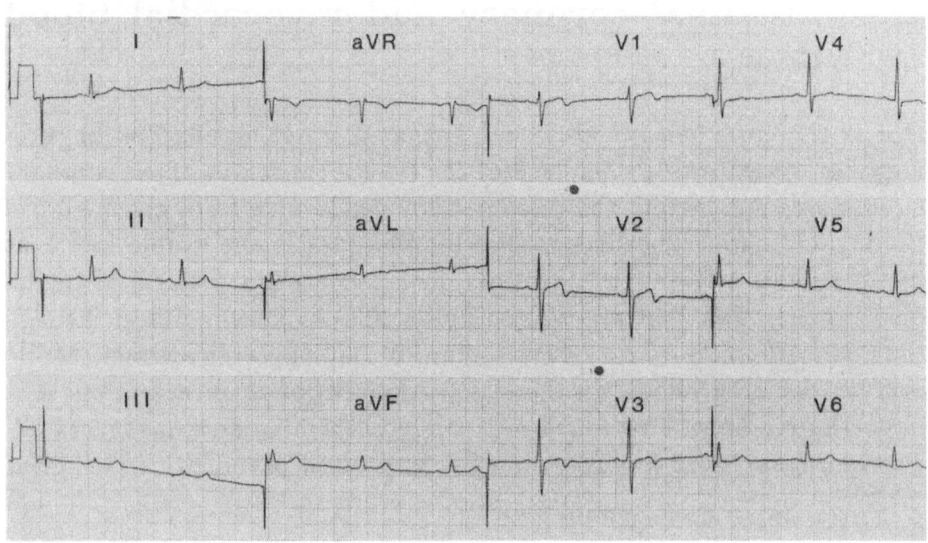

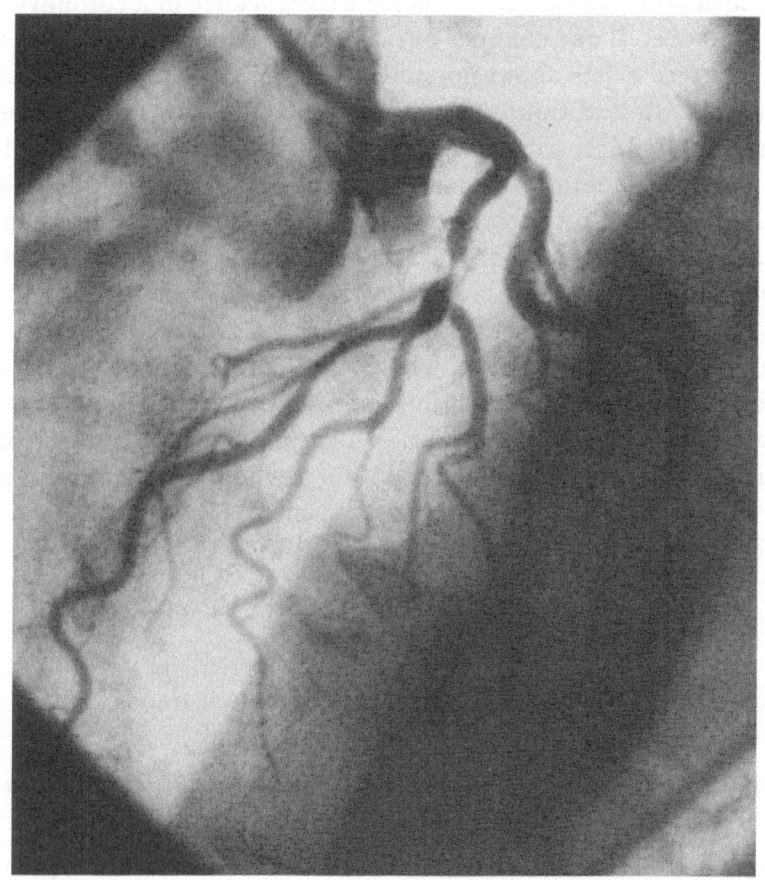

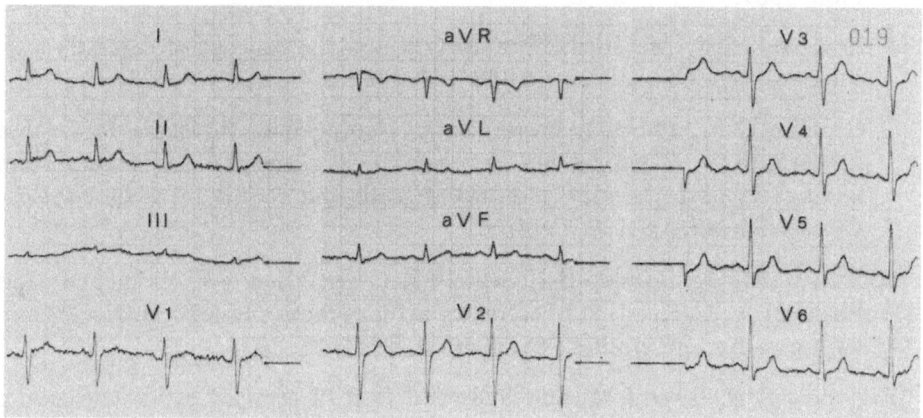

direct information about the physiologic significance of a coronary artery lesion. Moreover, if one confines oneself to measurement of maximal flow only, no concern exists about possible hyperemic effects of the measuring method itself. In addition, unlike CFR, maximal flow is not dependent on heart rate, left ventricular hypertrophy, previous myocardial infarction in other segments, previous PTCA, or other confounding factors. It is only dependent on pressure, which can easily be measured and corrected for [4, 34]. If, therefore, a reliable method would be available to assess maximal myocardial blood flow in conscious man during routine cardiac catheterization, this would greatly contribute to a better understanding of the physiologic significance of a coronary artery stenosis. In this book such a method is described using mean transit time of contrast passage as the relevant parameter. Unlike previous videodensitometric methods, no effort at all is made to obtain any information about resting flow or coronary flow reserve, but instead maximal flow will be assessed more accurately than before.

References

[1] Sones F M and Shirey E K. Cine coronary arteriography. *Mod Concepts Cardiov Dis*, 31:735–738, 1962.

[2] Judkins M P. Selective coronary arteriography. I. A percutaneous transfemoral technic. *Radiology*, 89:815–824, 1967.

[3] Klocke F J. Measurements of coronary flow reserve: defining pathophysiology versus making decisions about patient care. *Circulation*, 76:1183–1189, 1987.

[4] Hoffman J I E. Maximal coronary flow and the concept of coronary vascular reserve. *Circulation*, 70:153–159, 1984.

[5] Grondin C M, Dyrda I, Pasternac A, Campeau L, Bourassa M G, and Lesperance J. Discrepancies between cineangiography and postmortem findings in patients with coronary disease and recent revascularization. *Circulation*, 49:703–708, 1974.

[6] Hutchins G M, Bulkley B H, Ridolfi R L, Griffith L S C, Lohr F T, and Piasio M A. Correlation of coronary arteriograms and left ventriculogram with postmortem studies. *Circulation*, 56:32–37, 1977.

[7] Arnett E N, Isner J M, and Redwood D R. Coronary artery narrowing in coronary heart disease: comparison of cineangiographic and necropsy findings. *Ann Intern Med*, 91:350–356, 1979.

[8] Roberts W C and Jones A A. Quantitation of coronary arterial narrowing at necropsy in sudden coronary death. *Am J Cardiol*, 44:39–44, 1979.

[9] Isner J M, Kishel J, and Kent K M. Accuracy of angiographic determination of left main coronary arterial narrowing. *Circulation*, 63:1056–1061, 1981.

[10] Blankenhorn D H and Curry P J. The accuracy of arteriography and ultrasound imaging for atherosclerosis measurement: A review. *Arch Pathol Lab Med*, 106:483–490, 1982.

[11] Zir L M, Miller S W, Dinsmore R F, Gilbert J P, and Harthorne J W. Interobserver variability in coronary arteriography. *Circulation*, 53:627–632, 1976.

[12] Galbraith J E and Murphy M L Desoyza N. Coronary angiogram interpretation: Interobserver variability. *JAMA*, 240:2053–2059, 1981.

[13] Gould K L. Quantification of coronary artery stenosis in vivo. *Circul Res*, 57:341–353, 1985.

[14] White C W, Wright C B, Doty D B, Hiratza L F, Eastham C L, Harrison D G, and Marcus M L. Does visual interpretation of the coronary arteriogram predict the physiological importance of a coronary stenosis? *N Engl J Med*, 310:819–824, 1984.

[15] Harrison D G, White C W, Hiratzka L F, Doty D B Barnes D H, Eastham C L, and Marcus M L. The value of lesion cross-sectional area determined by quantitative coronary arteriography in assessing the physiologic significance of proximal left anterior descending coronary arterial stenoses. *Circulation*, 69:1111–1119, 1984.

[16] Nissen S E and Gurley J C. Assessment of the functional significance of coronary stenoses. Is digital angiography the answer? *Circulation*, 81:1431–1435, 1990.

[17] Van der Werf T. Coronary arteriography. In T van der Werf, editor, *Cardiovascular Pathophysiology*, pages 276–286. Oxford University Press, Oxford, 1980.

[18] Vlodaver Z, Frech R, Van Tassel R A, and Edwards J E. Correlation of the antemortem coronary arteriogram and the postmortem specimen. *Circulation*, 47:162–168, 1973.

[19] Pijls N H J. Meting van de doorbloeding van het myocard. *Cardioselecta*, 7:1–16, 1989.

[20] Fung Y C. Blood flow in arteries. In Y C Fung, editor, *Biodynamics, part II, Circulation*, pages 77–165. Springer, New York, 1984.

[21] Kirkeeide R L, Gould K L, and Parsel L. Assessment of coronary stenoses by myocardial perfusion imaging during pharmacologic coronary vasodilation. VIII. Validation of coronary flow reserve as a single integrated functional measure of stenosis severity reflecting all its geometric dimensions. *J Am Coll Cardiol*, 7:103–113, 1986.

[22] Gould K L, Kirkeeide R L, and Buchi M. Coronary flow reserve as a physiologic measure of stenosis severity. *J Am Coll Cardiol*, 15:459–474, 1990.

[23] Gould K L, Lipscomb K, and Hamilton G W. Physiologic basis for assessing critical coronary stenosis: instantaneous flow response and regional distribution during coronary hyperemia as measures of coronary flow reserve. *Am J Cardiol*, 33:87–94, 1974.

[24] Folts J D, Gallagher K, and Rowe G G. Hemodynamic effects of controlled degrees of coronary artery stenosis in short-term and long-term studies in dogs. *J Thorac Cardiov Surg*, 73:722–727, 1977.

[25] Young D F, Cholvin N R, and Roth A C. Flow in the major branches of the left coronary artery during experimental coronary insufficiency in the unanesthetized dog. *Circ Res*, 36:735–743, 1975.

[26] Marcus M L. Basic regulatory mechanisms in the coronary circulation. In M L Marcus, editor, *The coronary circulation in health and disease*, pages 93–112. McGraw-Hill, New York, 1983.

[27] Gerber K H and Higgins C B. Comparative effects of ionic and nonionic contrast materials on coronary and peripheral blood flow. *Invest Radiol*, 17:292–298, 1982.

[28] Schraeder R, Baller D, Hoeft A, Korb H, Wolpers H G, and Hellige G. Reduced side effects of low osmolality nonionic contrast media in coronary arteriography. In V Taenzer and E Zeitler, editors, *Contrast media in urography, angiography and computerized tomography*, pages 67–77. George Thieme Verlag, Stutgart, New York, 1983.

[29] Simon R, Koch M, Hermann G, Amende I, and Lichtlen P R. Direct effects of an ionic nonionic contrast agent on the coronary circulation in man. In *Proceedings Xth World Congress Cardiology*, page 294. Washington, 1986.

[30] Wilson R F, Laughlin D E, Ackell P H, Chilian W M, Holida M D, Hartley C J, Armstrong M L, Marcus M L, and White C W. Transluminal subselective measurement of coronary artery blood flow velocity and vasodilator reserve in man. *Circulation*, 72:82–92, 1985.

[31] Pijls N H J, Bos H S, Uijen G J H, and Van der Werf T. Is ionic isotonic iohexol the contrast agent of choice for quantitative myocardial videodensitometry? *Intern J Cardiac Imag*, 3:117–126, 1988.

[32] Pijls N H J, Uijen G J H, Hoevelaken A, Pijnenburg T, Van Leeuwen K, Fast J H, Bos J S, Aengevaeren W R M, and Van der Werf T. Mean transit time for videodensitometric assessment of myocardial perfusion and the concept of maximal flow ratio: A validation study in the intact dog and a pilot study in man. *Int J Cardiac Imag*, 5:191–202, 1990.

[33] O'Neill W W, Walton J A, Bates E R, Colfer H T, Aueron F M, LeFree M T, Pitt B, and Vogel R A. Criteria for successful coronary angioplasty as assessed by alterations in coronary vasodilatory reserve. *J Am Coll Cardiol*, 3:1382–1390, 1984.

[34] Zijlstra F, Den Boer A, Reiber J H C, Van Es G A, Lubsen J, and Serruys P W. Assessment of immediate and long-term results of percutaneous transluminal coronary angioplasty. *Circulation*, 78:15–24, 1988.

[35] Pijls N H J, Uijen G J H, Hoevelaken A, Arts T, Aengevaeren W R M, Bos H S, Fast J H, Van Leeuwen K L, and Van der Werf T. Mean transit time for the assessment of myocardial perfusion by videodensitometry. *Circulation*, 81:1331–1340, 1990.

Chapter 2

Methods of Measuring Myocardial Blood Flow

In this chapter, some methods will be described which have been developed to measure flow in the coronary circulation. Some of these methods are restricted to the animal laboratory or to the anesthetized patient during open heart surgery, some others can also be applied in conscious man. An overview of both groups is presented below.

2.1 Laboratory methods

Over time, many methods have been developed to measure blood flow in laboratory animals. Some of these methods provide direct information about myocardial perfusion, some of them measure flow through the large epicardial arteries which is considered to be representative for myocardial blood flow. Only those methods will be described which are either of historical value or are frequently used at present.

2.1.1 Timed venous collection

The earliest successful attempt to measure coronary blood flow in animals was performed by Langendorff almost one century ago by collecting coronary venous blood with a graduated cylinder and a stopwatch [1]. The method is called timed venous collection and is still used in some types of preparation, especially when the heart is either excised or exposed. This method can not be applied in the intact animal or in chronic experiments. Underestimation of flow occurs if too much blood drains into venous channels (e.g. Thebesian veins) not entering the coronary sinus. Despite these and a number of other limitations, the method has considerably contributed to the insights into the coronary circulation.

2.1.2   Electromagnetic flow measurement

The principle of electromagnetic (EM) flow measurement is based upon Faraday's law of induction: a magnetic field is applied perpendicular to the direction of blood flow. Blood is considered as a moving conductor in the magnetic field and produces an induced voltage, its magnitude being proportional to blood flow. Electromagnetic flow meters are routinely applied in the animal laboratory for over 30 years and enable accurate volumetric measurements of laminar and turbulent flow. The method integrates flow across the entire vessel. Its applicability, however, is restricted by a number of technical and methodological problems. Although the probes are not as bulky as in the earlier days, they are still quite heavy compared with Doppler probes and circular dissection of native coronary vessels remains necessary to place the probe firmly. The probes are rather expensive. Furthermore, determination of zero flow and calibration requires repeated attention and patience of the investigator. In acute experiments, vessel contact may be variable and may change with alternations in intravascular pressure or vascular diameter. If implanted chronically, the vessel contact improves by fibrous adhesions and the stability of the flow signal is improved. *If applied in a proper way, the method is considered as the gold standard for flow measurement in the animal laboratory.*

In humans, the application of EM flow measurement is restricted to the operating room for measuring flow in bypass grafts. These measurements, however, are difficult to interpret because adequate zero-ing and calibrating is hard and often neglected by lack of time, and because the size of the myocardium to be perfused is mostly undetermined.

2.1.3   Epicardial ultrasonic flow velocity measurement

When ultrasound waves, emitted by a piezo-electric crystal, hit moving erythrocytes, they will be reflected and the frequency of the reflected waves will be changed in a predictable way according to the Doppler equation:

$$f_d = 2f_0 \cdot \frac{v \cos \alpha}{c} \qquad (2.1)$$

where f_d represents the frequency shift, f_0 the frequency of the emitted waves, v the velocity of the erythrocytes, α the angle of the ultrasound waves with respect to the direction of motion of the erythrocytes and c the velocity of ultrasound in human blood (approximately 1500 m/s).

Using the Doppler principle, blood flow velocity in exposed coronary arteries can be measured accurately and used as a measure of coronary flow. The probes are very tiny and even can be applied superficially on the blood vessel [2]. If an epicardial circular probe is used, the angle α is well known (generally 45°) and remains constant. Furthermore, in the chronic experiment the diameter of the vessel is kept constant by the probe because of fibrous ingrowth. If using pulsed Doppler, one single crystal can be used for both emitting and receiving the signal and one can make sure that the highest velocity (mostly in the center of the vessel) is measured.

In many studies and under various conditions, changes in velocity have been correlated to changes in flow measured by timed venous collection, EM probes, and microspheres. In these studies the reliability of ring-mounted, epicardial Doppler probes to accurately reflect changes in volumetric flow has been repeatedly demonstrated [3, 4, 5, 6]. For the calculation of absolute flow, theoretically, the cross-sectional area of the vessel must be multiplied by the cross-sectionally averaged flow velocity. One should be careful, however, because only velocity at one point of the profile (usually the center) is measured and the profile is unknown. Therefore, flow calculated by Doppler is proportional to, but not necessarily equal to the actual flow. In the animal experiments as described in chapter 6 of this book, Doppler probes were used to assess changes in coronary flow in chronically instrumented dogs. Before sacrifice, in six dogs the Doppler probes were calibrated volumetrically against EM flow probes. An excellent correlation was present in all dogs ($r = 0.96 \pm 0.05$; mean ± SD) over a wide range of 0-250 ml/min [7]. An example of the result of one of these calibration experiments is shown in figure 2.1 and figure 2.2. The proportionality factor k varied from 1.1 to 1.7 in the six dogs and showed a relation with the vessel's diameter.

In contrast to the use of the Doppler catheter in human coronary arteries (cf section 2.2.3), epicardial Doppler flow velocity measurement can replace EM flow measurement if relative flow is required or if calibration is performed afterwards. Apart from the fact that the probes are light, small, and inexpensive, the method is easily applicable without concern about zero flow. Only fluids containing particles can be

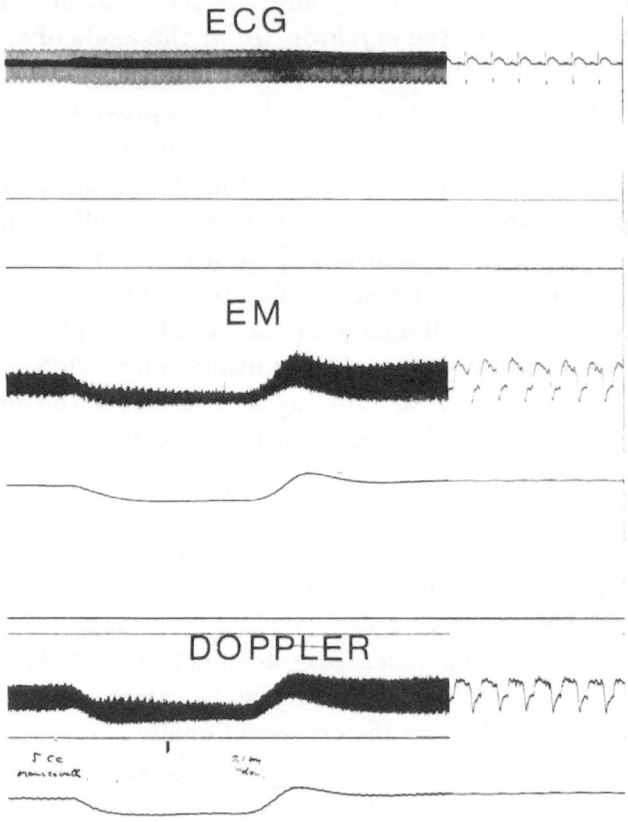

Figure 2.1: *Volumetric calibration of a ring-mounted, epicardial Doppler probe against an electromagnetic (EM) flow probe at the end of a chronic dog experiment. Phasic and mean tracings are displayed.*

measured. Besides their accuracy, two more advantages of EM as well as Doppler methods in comparison with other present methods, are the high frequency response and the unlimited number of measurements which can be performed.

2.1.4 Microspheres

Microspheres are small particles which are labeled in one or the other way to detect their distribution. These particles should have a size slightly larger than erythrocytes to effect capillary entrapment after in-

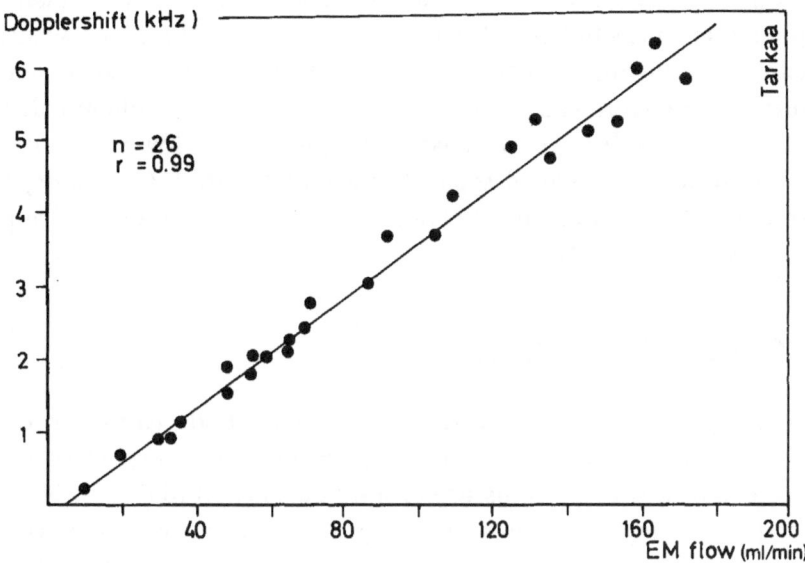

Figure 2.2: *Volumetric calibration of a ring-mounted, epicardial Doppler probe against an electromagnetic (EM) flow probe at the end of a chronic dog experiment. A linear relation between both measurements is present over a range of 0-200 ml/min being the range of canine circumflex flow.*

jection into the circulation. The distribution of microspheres in the different parts of the myocardium (or other organs) will reflect blood flow to these tissue segments [8]. In the assessment of the coronary circulation, mostly microspheres with a diameter of $15\mu m$ are used [9, 10]. The microspheres are usually injected into the left atrium to ensure adequate mixing [8, 11]. Calibration is performed by taking an arterial sample at a known flow rate at the time of microsphere injection [12, 13]. Myocardial flow is expressed as a ratio to this known flow rate.

Microspheres techniques are applied in a large number of animal models. Labelling is mostly provided by various gamma-emitting isotopes and microspheres can be detected by a gamma camera. Differential isotopes can be used and distinguished by spectroscopy [12]. In that case, a gamma counter is necessary to analyze tissue and blood samples following the death of the animal.

In contrast to the previous methods, the microsphere approach provides a direct measure of the perfusion of the myocardium itself. If microspheres are injected selectively, the perfusion field of a particular vessel can be delineated. Further advantages are that measurement of transmural distribution can be performed and that no significant disturbance of hemodynamics occurs. Disadvantages are the low frequency response, the limited number of separate measurements [14], microsphere loss if too much time is present between measurement and sacrifice [15], and exposure to radioactivity.

2.2   Clinical methods

In contrast to the sophisticated and accurate methods to measure myocardial perfusion in animals, current approaches of studying coronary and myocardial flow in humans are crude and only available in few laboratories [13]. They are either not very accurate, very expensive and laborious, or imply certain risks for the patient. Due to these limitations, knowledge about the coronary circulation in conscious man is far behind compared to the animal laboratory. Two remarks have to be made at this place.

1. In many situations, comparison of flow under different conditions provides more information about the functional status of the coronary circulation than does one single volumetric measurement. For example, coronary flow reserve as defined in section 2.1 is located in a well-defined range in normal individuals, independent of the absolute flow. In studying the effects of interventions, such as PTCA or long-lasting lipid lowering drug therapy, relative changes in flow are more important to evaluate the result than volumetric improvement [7]. This will be discussed in more detail in chapter 6 and 7.

2. Normal coronary flow, expressed as ml/min, varies considerably between different individuals and in different situations and therefore a volumetric value is not easily to interpret. The most physiologic approach would be to express perfusion as ml/min/100 g heart muscle and to specify other hemodynamic variables at the time of measurement. Measuring heart weight, however, seems to be utopian in intact man. For this reason it would be convenient if another parameter for "normal" coronary or myocardial flow could

be defined. Preferably, such a parameter should describe the functional status of the coronary vascular system and should not be dependent on changes in actual hemodynamic status, presence of left ventricular hypertrophy, or other pathological entities not affecting the vascular system itself. In the chapters 7 and 9, the value of mean transit time of contrast passage at maximal hyperemia is discussed for this purpose.

2.2.1 Coronary sinus thermodilution

Application of the thermodilution principle in the coronary sinus was introduced by Ganz [16]. A small catheter is introduced deeply into the coronary sinus and cold saline is delivered at its tip. Theoretically, flow can be calculated from the changes in blood temperature, registered by a thermistor close to the outlet of the coronary sinus. An advantage of this method is that only right heart catheterization is required. The disadvantages and limitations of the method, however, are numerous. Mixing of blood and indicator is often inadequate. Only a measure of the total flow through the left coronary artery is provided and no differentiation between different parts of the myocardium is possible. Data about perfusion of the right ventricular myocardium cannot be obtained. Because of the slow time constant inherent to this technique (several seconds), no phasic flow can be measured and a steady state has to be present, not disturbed by changes in heart rhythm or hemodynamic status. Finally, convincing validation studies have never been presented and it is assumed that only substantial changes in flow of approximately 25-30% can be measured accurately in man [4, 13, 17]. In the presence of coronary artery disease, the reliability is even worse [13].

2.2.2 Gas clearance methods

Just like thermodilution in the coronary sinus, these methods are based upon indicator dilution techniques. After administration of certain inert gasses by inhalation (He, Ar) or by direct intracoronary injection (^{133}Xe), extraction occurs by the myocardium. Therefore, a difference in concentration will be created between coronary arterial blood (saturated) and coronary venous blood. After ceasing the administration, a reverse phenomenon occurs (desaturation). Theoretically, myocardial perfusion can be calculated from the rate of administration and the concentration differences.

The practical limitations of this method are roughly comparable to the coronary sinus thermodilution method, while simultaneous blood samples from the coronary arterial and venous system have to be obtained [13]. Because of these limitations, none of these methods has found widespread clinical application.

2.2.3   The Doppler catheter

The Doppler catheter has been developed by Marcus and coworkers at the University of Iowa in the early eighties [18, 19, 20]. It is a tiny, 3-5 F catheter (Ø1.0-1.6 mm) with a crystal mounted on its top. After introduction of the catheter into a branch of the coronary arterial system, flow velocity can be measured both before and after a hyperemic stimulus [20]. The advantages of this method are the relative ease of use and the fact that selective measurements can be performed. As is the case with epicardial Doppler probes (cf section 2.1.3), the frequency response is excellent and phasic flow can be measured over time. In animal validation studies satisfactory results have been obtained. In clinical practice, however, results have been less uniform [18, 19, 21, 22, 23].

The method has a number of considerable disadvantages. Firstly, intracoronary manipulation is necessary and, just as is the case in angioplasty, implies a small, but definite risk of damage to the coronary arteries [18]. If a stenosis is present in the proximal part of a branch or just beyond a side branch, the catheter has to pass the lesion before reliable measurements can be performed. This can result in further obstruction at the site of the lesion by the catheter itself and will result in overestimation of functional severity of the stenosis. The same problem occurs if the catheter is introduced in small vessels with a cross-sectional area of less than $2.5mm^2$ [20, 23]. Furthermore, the tip of the catheter is floating freely and cannot be stabilized in the center of the vessel. Because the distribution of velocities in a cross-sectional area is unknown, may unpredictably be disturbed by the catheter itself, and may change by interventions, it is not clear if comparable velocities are measured before and after such an intervention [23, 24]. Moreover, unlike in the case of an epicardial ring-mounted Doppler probe, in which case the diameter of the vessel is fixed, changes in vessel diameter may occur up to 20% (corresponding with area variations up to 40%), thus affecting the reliability of velocity to predict flow [25]. The latter problem can be circumvented by previous administration of nitroglycerine [26], but this in turn limits the applicability of the methods in the diagnosis of some pathologic states as for example diseases accompanied by increased coronary vasomotor tone.

Despite these limitations, the Doppler catheter has constituted a valuable addition to the study of the coronary circulation in normal and pathologic situations.

2.2.4 Videodensitometry

After injection of contrast agent into a coronary artery, temporal changes in contrast density of the myocardium can be studied and used to calculate flow according to the indicator dilution theory. Although the principles of this method have been suggested by Rutishauser almost 25 years ago [27, 28, 29], until now no physiologically sound and reliable clinical application has been possible [30]. In this book a new videodensitometric approach is described, enabling accurate measurement of the maximal flow achievable through almost every arbitrary part of the myocardium. The theory of flow calculation by videodensitometry, its advantages and limitations, and a historical overview of previous attempts to use this method for flow measurement in a clinically useful way, are described extensively in chapter 3 and 4.

2.2.5 Positron emission tomography

After its introduction in the late seventies [31, 32], positron emission tomography (PET) has been considered for a long time as an expensive research method with little clinical utility [22]. After intravenous or intra-arterial administration of positron emitting isotopes (^{13}N-ammonia, ^{82}Rb), these are extracted by tissues, e.g. the myocardium, and the distribution of the positron emitting isotopes can be detected by a positron camera. If ^{82}Rb is used, the first pass flow of the tracer through the left ventricular cavity can be measured and considered as the arterial input function, necessary for quantitative myocardial flow measurement [33].

The great advantage of this method is that it provides a powerful approach permitting repeated measurements of the regional distribution of coronary blood flow in awake humans. A disadvantage is that the equipment is very expensive. A positron camera, and in the original approach a cyclotron for generating positron emitting isotopes, are needed. In more recent approaches the cyclotron can be replaced by a less expensive ^{82}Rb generator [33]. During the last years, a number of studies has been performed, especially by the University of Texas group, to transform the method towards an economically and practically feasible test for diagnosis of symptomatic and asymptomatic coronary artery disease [33, 34]. Further investigation of this promising technique is mandatory and is still in progress.

2.2.6   Other methods

A number of other methods for coronary or myocardial flow assessment is currently under investigation. These include ultrafast computed tomography (ultrafast CT), (ultrafast CT) magnetic resonance imaging (MRI), (MRI) and contrast echocardiography. These methods will not be discussed in detail. They share the theoretical advantage that flow information can be obtained from different layers of the myocardium, i.e. the transmural distribution of flow can theoretically be measured. This would be useful because coronary artery disease initially often results in a decrease of subendocardial perfusion. To this date, too little data are known to have a clear judgement about the future value of these methods.

References

[1] Langendorff O.   Untersuchungen am ueberlebenden Saugetierherzen. *Pfluegers Arch Physiol*, 61:291–332, 1895.

[2] Marcus M, Wright C, Doty D, Eastham C, Laughlin D, Krumm P, Fastenow C, and Brody M. Measurements of coronary velocity and reactive hyperemia in the coronary circulation of humans. *Circ Res*, 49:877–891, 1981.

[3] Vatner S F, Franklin D, and Vancitters R L. Simultaneous comparison and calibration of the Doppler and electromagnetic flowmeters. *J Appl Physiol*, 29:907–910, 1970.

[4] Hartley C J and Cole J S. An ultrasonic pulsed Doppler system for measuring blood flow in small vessels. *J Appl Physiol*, 37:626–629, 1974.

[5] Haywood J R, Shaffer R A, Fastenow C, Fink G D, and Brody M J. Regional blood flow measurement with pulsed Doppler flowmeter in conscious rat. *Am J Physiol*, 241:H273–H278, 1981.

[6] Van Orden D E, Farley D B, Fastenow C, and Brody M J. A technique for monitoring blood flow changes with miniaturized Doppler flow probes. *Am J Physiol*, 247:H1005–H1009, 1984.

[7] Pijls N H J, Uijen G J H, Hoevelaken A, Arts T, Aengevaeren W R M, Bos H S, Fast J H, Van Leeuwen K L, and Van der Werf T. Mean transit time for the assessment of myocardial perfusion by videodensitometry. *Circulation*, 81:1331–1340, 1990.

[8] Buckberg G D, Luck J C, Payne D B, Hoffman J I E, Utley J R, and Carlson E L. Measurement of cardiac output with an organ trapping of radioactive microspheres. *J Appl Physiol*, 31:598–612, 1971.

[9] Yipintsol T, Dobbs W A, Scanlon P D, Knopp T J, and Bassingthwaighte J B. Regional distribution of diffusible tracers and carbonized microspheres in the left ventricle of isolated dog hearts. *Circ Res*, 33:573–578, 1973.

[10] Tripp M R, Meyer M W, Einzig S, Leonard J J, Swayze C R, and Fox I J. Simultaneous regional myocardial blood flows by tritiated water and microspheres. *Am J Physiol*, 232:H173–H180, 1977.

[11] Marcus M L, Heistad D D, Ehrhardt J C, and Abboud F M. Total and regional cerebral blood flow measurement with 7-, 10-, 15-, 25- and 50-μm microspheres. *J Appl Physiol*, 35:148–158, 1973.

[12] Makowski E L, Meschia G, Droegemueller W, and Battaglia F C. Measurement of umbilical arterial blood flow to the sheep placenta and fetus in utero: Distribution to cotyledons and the intercotyledonary chorion. *Circ Res*, 21:163–175, 1967.

[13] Marcus M L and White C W Wilson R F. Methods of measurement of myocardial blood flow in patients: a critical review. *Circulation*, 76:245–252, 1987.

[14] Baer R W, Verrier E D, Vlahakes G J, Payne B D, and Hoffman J I E. Validation of eight sequential myocardial blood flow determinations with radioactive microspheres using least- squares analysis. *Circulation, suppl 3*, 62:65, 1980.

[15] Murdock R H and Cobb F R. Effects of infarcted myocardium on regional blood flow measurements to ischemic regions in canine heart. *Circ Res*, 47:701–709, 1980.

[16] Ganz W, Donoso R Tamura K, Marcus H S, Yoshiola S, and Swan H J C. Measurement of coronary sinus blood flow by continuous thermodilution in man. *Circulation*, 44:181–195, 1971.

[17] Marcus M L. Autoregulation in the coronary circulation. pages 93–112. McGraw-Hill, New York, 1983.

[18] Wilson R F, Laughlin D E, Ackell P H, Chilian W M, Holida M D, Hartley C J, Armstrong M L, Marcus M L, and White C W. Transluminal subselective measurement of coronary artery blood flow velocity and vasodilator reserve in man. *Circulation*, 72:82–92, 1985.

[19] Sibley D H, Millar H D, Hartley C J, and Whitlow P L. Subselective measurement of coronary blood flow velocity using a steerable Doppler catheter. *J Am Coll Cardiol*, 8:1332–1340, 1986.

[20] Wilson R F, Marcus M L, and White C W. Prediction of the physiologic significance of coronary arterial lesions by quantitative lesion geometry in patients with limited coronary artery disease. *Circulation*, 75:723–732, 1987.

[21] Klocke F J. Measurements of coronary flow reserve: defining pathophysiology versus making decisions about patient care. *Circulation*, 76:1183–1189, 1987.

[22] Harrison D G, White C W, Hiratzka L F, Doty D B Barnes D H, Eastham C L, and Marcus M L. The value of lesion cross-sectional area determined by quantitative coronary arteriography in assessing the physiologic significance of proximal left anterior descending coronary arterial stenoses. *Circulation*, 69:1111–1119, 1984.

[23] Serruys P W, Juilliere Y, Zijlstra F, Beatt K J, De Feyter P J, Suryapranata H, Van den Brand M, and Roelandt J. Coronary blood flow velocity during percutaneous transluminal coronary angioplasty as a guide for assessment of the functional result. *Am J Cardiol*, 61:253–259, 1988.

[24] Kilpatrick D and Webber S B. Intravascular blood velocity in simulated coronary artery stenoses. *Cathet Cardiovasc Diagn*, 12:317–323, 1986.

[25] Gould K L. Functional measures of coronary stenosis severity at cardiac catheterization. *J Am Coll Cardiol*, 16:198–199, 1990.

[26] Jost S, Rafflenbeul W, Reil G H, Trappe H J, Gulba D, Hecker H, Gerhardt U, and Knop I. Elimination of variable vasomotor tone in studies with repeated quantitative coronary angiography. *J Am Coll Cardiol (in press)*, 1990.

[27] Rutishauser W, Simon H, Stucky J P, Schad N, Noseda G, and Wellauer J. Evaluation of roentgen cinedensitometry for flow measurement in models and in the intact circulation. *Circulation*, 36:951–963, 1967.

[28] Rutishauser W, Bussmann W D, Noseda G, Meier W, and Wellauer J. Blood flow measurement through single coronary arteries by roentgen densitometry. part I: A comparison of flow measured by a radiologic technique applicable in the intact organism and by electromagnetic flowmeter. *Am J Roentgenol*, 109:12–20, 1970.

[29] Rutishauser W, Noseda G, Bussman W D, and Preter B. Blood flow measurement through single coronary arteries by roentgen densitometry. Part II: Right coronary artery flow in conscious man. *Am J Roentgenol*, 109:21–24, 1970.

[30] Nissen S E and Gurley J C. Assessment of the functional significance of coronary stenoses. Is digital angiography the answer? *Circulation*, 81:1431–1435, 1990.

[31] Schelbert H R, Phelps M E, Hoffman E J, Huang S C, Selin C E, and Kuhl D E. Regional myocardial perfusion assessed with n-13 labeled ammonia and positron emission computerized axial tomography. *Am J Cardiol*, 43:209–218, 1979.

[32] Gould K L, Schelbert H, Phelps M, and Hoffman E. Noninvasive assessment of coronary stenoses by myocardial perfusion imaging during pharmacologic coronary vasodilation. V. Detection of 47% diameter coronary stenosis with intravenous [13]nh and emission computed tomography in intact dogs. *Am J Cardiol*, 43:200–208, 1979.

[33] Gould K L, Goldstein R A, Mullani N A, Kirkeeide R L, Wong W-H, Tewson T J, Berridge M S, Bolomey L A, Hartz R K, Smalling R W, Fuentes F, and Nishikawa A. Noninvasive assessment of coronary stenoses by myocardial perfusion imaging during pharmacologic coronary vasodilation. VIII. Clinical feasibility of positron cardiac imaging without a cyclotron using generator-produced rubidium-82. *J Am Coll Cardiol*, 7:775–789, 1986.

[34] Gould K L. Identifying and measuring severity of coronary artery stenosis. Quantitative coronary arteriography and positron emission tomography. *Circulation*, 78:237–245, 1988.

Chapter 3

Application of Indicator Dilution Theory in the Investigation of the Cardiovascular System

3.1 History

The earliest application of indicator dilution theory in the investigation of the cardiovascular system, was performed by Hering in 1829 [1]. Potassium ferrocyanide was injected intravenously and blood was collected from the contralateral vein. These blood samples were tested for ferrocyanide by adding ferric chloride. The first sample in which the Prussian blue reaction occurred, was considered by Hering as the blood which had completed the circuit from the vein to the right heart side, the pulmonary bed, the left heart side, the arterial system, and to the vein again. What Hering measured, in fact, was a kind of appearance time.

At the end of the 19th century, the method was improved by Stewart in a number of steps [2, 3, 4, 5]. One of the femoral arteries of Stewart's dogs was dissected free and placed over two electrodes so that the blood vessel formed one arm of a Wheatstone bridge. After introducing a tube in the carotid artery of the dogs, Stewart added a known amount and concentration of NaCl solution to the blood in the left ventricle of the heart for a number of seconds. A sample of the mixture of blood and saline was taken from the femoral artery, where its arrival was detected by a telephone howl which signaled the change in electrical resistance. The resistance of this blood sample was compared with a number of well-known dilutions of saline in blood. This, in fact, was a determina-

27

tion of the concentration of indicator in the arterial sample. Because the amount of indicator, injected per unit of time, as well as the concentration of saline in the femoral artery sample was known, flow could be calculated as the ratio of these two. Thirty years later, the method was further improved by Hamilton [6, 7, 8, 9], who used dye as indicator, which, bound to plasma proteins, did not pass out of the cardiovascular system during the period over which flow was measured.

All of the experiments described above, refer to laboratory animals and to the systemic circulation. In the fifties and sixties of this century, a number of methods has been developed to use indicator dilution theory for measurements of cardiac output in man, using several indicators such as indocyanine green or cold saline. When indocyanine green is used, a bolus of this dye is rapidly injected into the pulmonary artery and its appearance and concentration are recorded from a peripheral artery by a spectrophotometer.

More elegant is the thermodilution method, which was firstly applied in man by Van der Werf in 1965 [10] and widely popularized by Swan and coworkers between 1965 and 1972 [11, 12, 13, 14]. This technique can be performed repeatedly without accumulation of indicator and without recirculation problems.

All these techniques have in common that the amount of injected indicator has to be known exactly, which makes these methods hard to apply for flow measurement in the coronary circulation, using contrast agent as the indicator. For assessment of coronary flow, the theory of indicator dilution has to be extended in a way suggested by Rutishauser et al in the late sixties [15, 16, 17], avoiding the necessity of knowledge about the amount of injected indicator. Because familiarity with this latter, less well-known part of indicator dilution theory is indispensable for the understanding of the next chapters of this book, the theory will be outlined comprehensively below. For a more extensive review of this theory, we refer to the excellent work of Zierler in the Handbook of Physiology [18].

3.2   The two approaches in indicator dilution theory

In this section we will restrict ourselves to those situations in which a certain amount of indicator is rapidly injected - as a bolus - in a very

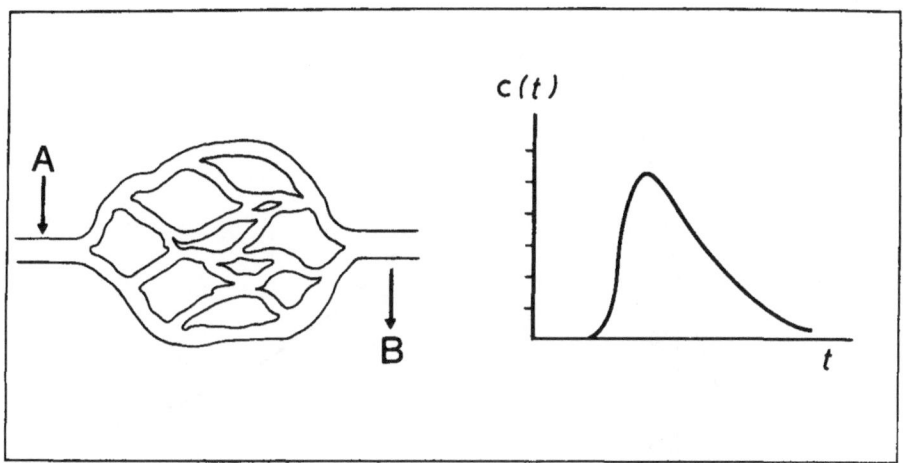

Figure 3.1: *After injection of indicator into a vascular network at site A, the passage of the indicator at site B can be represented by the concentration-time curve c(t), which is called the indicator dilution curve at B.*

short time: instantaneous injection of the indicator.

3.2.1 Measurement of Flow

Suppose that the flow through a branching vascular bed is constant and equals F, and that a certain well-known amount M of indicator is injected into this bed at site A (figure 3.1). After some time, the first particles of indicator will arrive at the measuring site B. The concentration of indicator at B, called $c(t)$, will increase for some time, reach a peak and decrease again. The graphic representation of indicator concentration as a function of time is called the indicator dilution curve.

Consider M as a large number of indicator particles (or molecules). The number of particles passing at B during the time interval Δt, between t_i and t_{i+1}, equals the number of particles passing per unit of time, multiplied by the length of the time interval, in other words: $c(t_i) \cdot F \cdot \Delta t$ (figure 3.2)

Because all particles pass at B between $t = 0$ and $t = \infty$, this mean that:

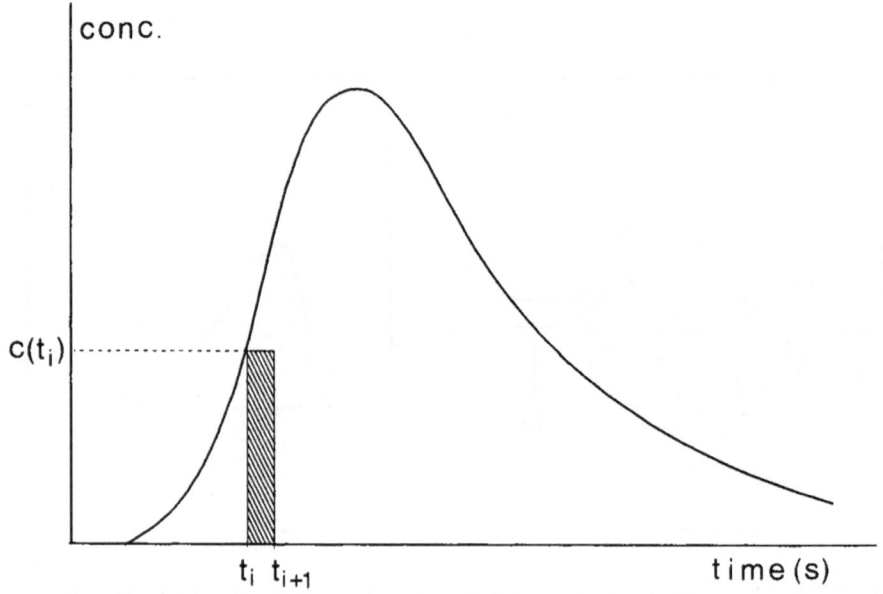

Figure 3.2: *Calculation of flow from the indicator dilution curve.*

$$M = \lim_{\Delta t \to 0} \sum_{i=0}^{\infty} (c(t_i) \cdot F \cdot \Delta t) \qquad (3.1)$$

or

$$M = \int_0^{\infty} c(t) \cdot F \cdot dt \qquad (3.2)$$

or

$$F = \frac{M}{\int_0^{\infty} c(t) \cdot dt} \qquad (3.3)$$

and it is this last expression which is used in most methods to calculate systemic flow as outlined above. *Essential features of this approach are that the amount M of injected indicator should be known whereas no knowledge about the volume of the vascular compartment is needed.*

3.2.2 Measurement of Volume

The calculation of volume is more complex. For this purpose, the function $h(t)$ is introduced which is defined as the fraction of indicator, passing per unit of time at site B at time t. In other words, $h(t)$ is the distribution function of transit times of the indicator particles. If it is assumed that flow of the indicator is representative for flow of the total fluid (complete mixing), $h(t)$ is also the distribution function of transit times of all fluid particles. Suppose that the total volume of fluid is made up of a very large number of volume elements dV_i which are defined in such a way that dV_i contains all fluid particles, present in the system at $t = 0$, with transit times between t_i and t_{i+1}. The fraction of fluid particles requiring times between t_i and t_{i+1} to pass at B, is $h(t_i) \cdot \Delta t$ by definition, and because the rate at which all fluid particles pass at B, equals F, the rate at which the particles making up dV_i pass at B, is $F \cdot h(t_i) \cdot \Delta t$. The total volume of dV_i equals the time t_i, required for all particles in dV_i to pass at B, multiplied by the rate at which they leave. In other words:

$$dV_i = t_i \cdot F \cdot h(t_i) \cdot \Delta t \qquad (3.4)$$

and by integration:

$$V = F \int_0^\infty t \cdot h(t) \cdot dt \qquad (3.5)$$

Because $h(t)$ is the distribution function of transit times, $\int_0^\infty t \cdot h(t) \cdot dt$ represents the mean transit time or mean circulation time T_{mn}, which is the average time, needed by one particle of indicator to travel from A to B. Therefore:

$$V = F \cdot T_{mn} \qquad (3.6)$$

or:

$$F = V/T_{mn} \qquad (3.7)$$

which states the fundamental fact that flow equals volume divided by mean transit time.

Essential features of this approach are, that no information is needed about the amount of indicator, injected at time = 0, whereas the volume of the vascular compartment should be known to calculate flow.

3.2.3   Calculation of Mean Transit Time

Mean transit time (T_{mn}) can now be calculated easily from the indicator dilution curve in the following way. When looking at the hatched rectangle in figure 3.2, it can be seen that the number of indicator particles, passing at B between t_i and t_{i+1}, equals the number of particles $c(t_i) \cdot F$ passing per unit of time, multiplied by the length of the time interval, Δt, in other words: $c(t_i) \cdot F \cdot \Delta t$. Therefore, the total (summed) transit time of all these indicator particles together equals $t_i \cdot c(t_i) \cdot F \cdot \Delta t$. The total transit time of all indicator particles together, by integration, is equal to

$$\int_0^\infty t \cdot c(t) \cdot F \cdot dt \tag{3.8}$$

and the mean transit time of the indicator particles can be obtained by dividing equation (3.8) by the total number of particles M, resulting in:

$$T_{mn} = \frac{\int_0^\infty t \cdot c(t) \cdot F \cdot dt}{M} \tag{3.9}$$

or

$$T_{mn} = \frac{F}{M} \int_0^\infty t \cdot c(t) \cdot dt \tag{3.10}$$

By substitution of equation (3.3) in (3.10), T_{mn} is obtained:

$$T_{mn} = \frac{\int_0^\infty t \cdot c(t) \cdot dt}{\int_0^\infty c(t) \cdot dt} \tag{3.11}$$

Equation (3.11) describes how mean transit time T_{mn} can be calculated from the indicator dilution curve $c(t)$. Because in the assessment of myocardial perfusion, using contrast agent as the indicator, the amount of injected contrast agent is unknown and changing because of the necessary leakage of the contrast agent back into the aorta and the unknown and changing distribution of contrast agent over the different branches of the coronary arterial tree, use of T_{mn} is advantageous because no knowledge about the amount of injected indicator is necessary. The characteristics of both approaches in indicator dilution theory are summarized in table 3.1.

Table 3.1: *Major approaches in indicator dilution theory.*

$F = M/ \int_0^\infty c(t)dt$	$F = V/T_{mn}$
• amount M of injected indicator should be known	• independent of the amount of injected indicator
• no information about vascular volume needed	• vascular volume V should be known

3.3 Videodensitometry and digital arteriography for flow assessment in the coronary circulation

Use of the principles as outlined above for the calculation of flow in the coronary system, using contrast agent as indicator and studying the passage of contrast as a function of time as an equivalent of the indicator dilution curve, was firstly suggested by Rutishauser [15, 16, 17]. In his approach, mean transit time of a contrast bolus through a measured length and diameter of a coronary arterial segment was determined by densitometry and used to calculate flow. Shortly thereafter, Robb et al. showed that visualization of contrast passage through the myocardium could be enhanced considerably by ECG-triggered subtraction imaging [19], and it was suggested that myocardial flow could be calculated by studying the temporal changes in contrast density in a myocardial region of interest: the time-density curve (figure 4.1). Analysis of these changes in contrast density, delineation of the time-density curves and subsequent calculation of time parameters from this curve (such as mean transit time) is referred to as *videodensitometry*, a definition already introduced by Wood in 1964 [20]. If digital methods are used for this purpose, also the term *digital radiography* is applied [21].

In the last decade many attempts have been made by a number of investigators to obtain reliable information about coronary flow and myocardial perfusion by videodensitometry in the intact man [22] - [34], but none of these attempts has resulted in an easily applicable method for the acquisition of reliable and reproducible flow data. Reasons for these disappointing results are a number of technical and methodological problems, which will be discussed in the next chapter.

References

[1] Hering E. Versuche, die Schnelligkeit des Blutlaufs und der Absonderung zu bestimmen. *Ztschr Physiol*, 3:85–98, 1829.

[2] Stewart G N. Researches on the circulation time in organs and on the influences which affect it. Part I-III. *J Physiol*, 15:1–62, 1893.

[3] Stewart G N. Researches on the circulation time in organs and on the influences which affect it. IV. The output of the heart. *J Physiol*, 22:159–183, 1898.

[4] Stewart G N. The output of the heart in dogs. *Am J Physiol*, 57:27–47, 1921.

[5] Stewart G N. The pulmonary circulation time, the quantity of blood in the lungs and the output of the heart. *Am J Physiol*, 58:20–38, 1921.

[6] Moore J W, Kinsman J M, Hamilton W F, and Spurling G R. Studies on the circulation. II. Cardiac output determinations; comparison of the injection method with the direct Fick procedure. *Am J Physiol*, 89:331–348, 1929.

[7] Hamilton W F, Moore J W, Kinsman J M, and Spurling R G. Studies on the circulation. IV. Further analysis of the injection method and of changes in hemodynamics under physiological and pathological conditions. *Am J Physiol*, 99:534–561, 1932.

[8] Hamilton W F and Remington J W. Comparison of the time concentration curves in arterial blood of diffusible and nondiffusible substances when injected at a constant rate and when injected instantaneously. *Am J Physiol*, 148:35–56, 1947.

[9] Meier P and Zierler K L. On the theory of the indicator-dilution method for measurement of blood flow and volume. *J Appl Physiol*, 6:731–734, 1954.

[10] Van der Werf T. De thermodilutiemethoden. In T van der Werf, editor, *Directe en indirecte stroommeting in het hart en de grote bloedvaten*, pages 130–139. Van Gorcum & Co, Assen, 1965.

[11] Rahimtoola S H and Swan H J C. Calculation of cardiac output from indicator dilution curves in the presence of mitral regurgitation. *Circulation*, 31:711–722, 1965.

[12] Shepherd R L, Higgs L M, and Glancy D L. Comparison of left ventricular and pulmonary arterial injection sites in determination of cardiac output by the indicator dilution technique. *Chest*, 62:175–179, 1972.

[13] Branthwaite M A and Bradley R D. Measurement of cardiac output by thermodilution in man. *J Appl Physiol*, 24:434–444, 1968.

[14] Ganz W, Donoso R, Marcus H S, Forrester J S, and Swan H J C. A new technique for measurement of cardiac output by thermodilution in man. *Amer J Cardiol*, 27:392–403, 1971.

[15] Rutishauser W, Simon H, Stucky J P, Schad N, Noseda G, and Wellauer J. Evaluation of roentgen cinedensitometry for flow measurement in models and in the intact circulation. *Circulation*, 36:951–963, 1967.

[16] Rutishauser W, Bussmann W D, Noseda G, Meier W, and Wellauer J. Blood flow measurement through single coronary arteries by roentgen densitometry. part I: A comparison of flow measured by a radiologic technique applicable in the intact organism and by electromagnetic flowmeter. *Am J Roentgenol*, 109:12–20, 1970.

[17] Rutishauser W, Noseda G, Bussman W D, and Preter B. Blood flow measurement through single coronary arteries by roentgen densitometry. Part II: Right coronary artery flow in conscious man. *Am J Roentgenol*, 109:21–24, 1970.

[18] Zierler K L. *Circulation times and the theory of indicator dilution methods for determining blood flow and volume*, pages 585–615. American Physiological Society, Washington DC, 1962.

[19] Robb R A, Wood E H, Ritman E L, Johnson S A, Sturm R E, Greenleaf J F, Gilbert B K, and Chevalier P A. Three-dimensional reconstruction and display of the working canine heart and lungs by multiplanar x-ray scanning videodensitometry. In *Computers in Cardiology 1974*, pages 151–163. IEEE Computer Society, Long Beach, 1974.

[20] Wood E H, Sturm R E, and Sanders J J. Data processing in cardiovascular physiology with particular reference to roentgen videodensitometry. *Mayo Clin Proc*, 39:849–865, 1964.

[21] Foerster J M, Link D P, Lanz B M T, Holcroft J W, and Mason D T. Measurement of coronary reactive hyperemia during clinical angiography by video dilution technique. *Acta Radiol Diag*, 22:209–216, 1981.

[22] Vogel R A and Mancini G B J. Assessment of coronary flow and myocardial perfusion with digital radiography. In G B J Mancini, editor, *Clinical applications of cardiac digital angiography*, pages 281–290. Raven Press, New York, 1988.

[23] Vogel R, LeFree M, Bates E, O'Neill W, Foster R, Kirlin P, Smith D, and Pitt B. Application of digital techniques to selective coronary arteriography: use of myocardial appearance time to measure coronary flow reserve. *Am Heart J*, 107:153–164, 1984.

[24] Vogel R A, Bates E R, O'Neill W W, Aueron F M, Meier B, and Gruentzig A R. Coronary flow reserve measured during cardiac catheterization. *Arch Intern Med*, 144:1773–1776, 1984.

[25] Hodgson J M, Legrand V, Bates E R, Mancini G B J, Aueron F M, O'Neill W W, Simon S B, Beauman G J, LeFree M T, and Vogel R A. Validation in dogs of a rapid digital angiographic technique to measure relative coronary blood flow during routine cardiac catheterization. *Am J Cardiol*, 55:188–193, 1985.

[26] Vogel R A. Radiographic assessment of coronary blood flow parameters. *Circulation*, 72:460–465, 1985.

[27] Cusma J T, Toggart E J, Folts J D, Peppler W W, Hagiandreou N J, Lee C S, and Mistretta C A. Digital subtraction imaging of coronary flow reserve. *Circulation*, 75:461–472, 1987.

[28] Zijlstra F, Den Boer A, Reiber J H C, Van Es G A, Lubsen J, and Serruys P W. Assessment of immediate and long-term results of percutaneous transluminal coronary angioplasty. *Circulation*, 78:15–24, 1988.

[29] Spiller P, Schmiel F K, Politz B, Block M, Fermor U, Hackbarth W, Jehle J, Korfer R, and Pannek H. Measurement of systolic and diastolic flow rates in the coronary artery system by x-ray videodensitometry. *Circulation*, 68:337–347, 1983.

[30] Ikeda H, Koga Y, Utsu F, and Toshima H. Quantitative evaluation of regional myocardial blood flow by videodensitometric analysis of digital subtraction coronary arteriography in humans. *J Am Coll Cardiol*, 8:809–816, 1986.

[31] Nissen S E, Elion J L, Booth D C, Evans J, and DeMaria A N. Value and limitations of computer analysis of digital subtraction angiography in the assessment of coronary flow reserve. *Circulation*, 73:562–571, 1986.

[32] Whiting J S, Drury J K, Pfaff J M, Chang B L, Eigler N L, Meerbaum S, Corday E, Nivatpumin T, Forrester J S, and Swan H J C. Digital angiographic measurement of radiographic contrast material kinetics for estimation of myocardial perfusion. *Circulation*, 73:789–798, 1986.

[33] Toggart E J and Mistretta C A. Digital coronary angiography: approaches using intravenous and direct methods. In G B J Mancini, editor, *Clinical applications of cardiac digital angiography*, pages 253–279. Raven Press, New York, 1988.

[34] Nissen S E and Gurley J C. Assessment of the functional significance of coronary stenoses. is digital angiography the answer? *Circulation*, 81:1431–1435, 1990.

Chapter 4

Problems and Limitations in the Application of Videodensitometry to Assess Coronary Blood Flow and Myocardial Perfusion

As discussed in the former chapter, a number of efforts have been made to use indicator dilution theory to calculate flow through the coronary circulation. For this purpose, the situation illustrated in figure 3.1, is translated to the vascular bed of the heart. This means that the injection site of the indicator corresponds with the tip of the catheter at the entrance of the left or the right coronary artery, whereas the measuring site is constituted by a so-called region of interest (ROI), placed over the part of the myocardium which should be investigated (figure 4.1). Application of the theory of chapter 3 to the coronary circulation, implies some simplifications which should be remarked: If the term 'constant flow' is used, mean flow (averaged over one heart cycle) is intended without taking into account the phasic (pulsatile) character of flow. Furthermore, in animal or man recirculation of contrast agent is expected. Because in clinical practice recirculation does not occur before data acquisition has been completed, this point will not be discussed extensively.

Four serious problems have to be solved, however, before calculation of flow can be performed by studying contrast agent passage. These problems are discussed below.

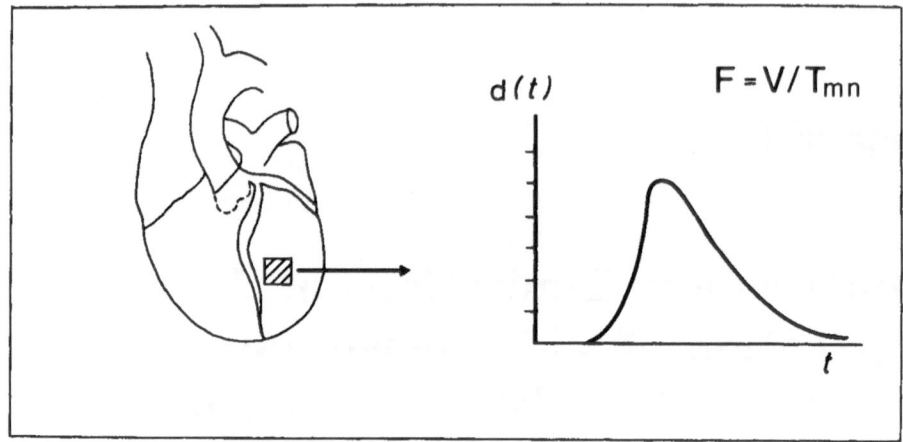

Figure 4.1: *Application of indicator dilution theory to assess myocardial blood flow by studying contrast passage (cf figure 3.1).*

4.1   Influence of the contrast agent on flow

From many investigations it is well known that injection of contrast agent into a coronary artery, after an initial short dip, is rapidly followed by a considerable increase in flow. The flow reaches a peak after approximately 8-10 seconds and returns to its baseline value after 30-60 seconds [1, 2, 3, 4, 5]. This is illustrated in figure 4.2, showing the hyperemic response in the left circumflex artery of a dog after injection of 6 ml of the contrast agents diatrizoate-370 and iohexol-140, respectively.

The increase in flow varies between 150 and 400% of the baseline value and is dependent on the type, concentration, injection rate, and amount of the contrast agent used [1, 2, 3, 4, 5]. Even in the most favorable circumstances, using the "least hyperemic" contrast agent in the lowest dose still enabling visualization of the myocardium, increases in flow of at least 50% are encountered (cf. appendix A). *This means that the parameter to be measured (flow) is influenced by the indicator itself (contrast agent), which is an unacceptable violation of the basic principles of indicator dilution theory.*

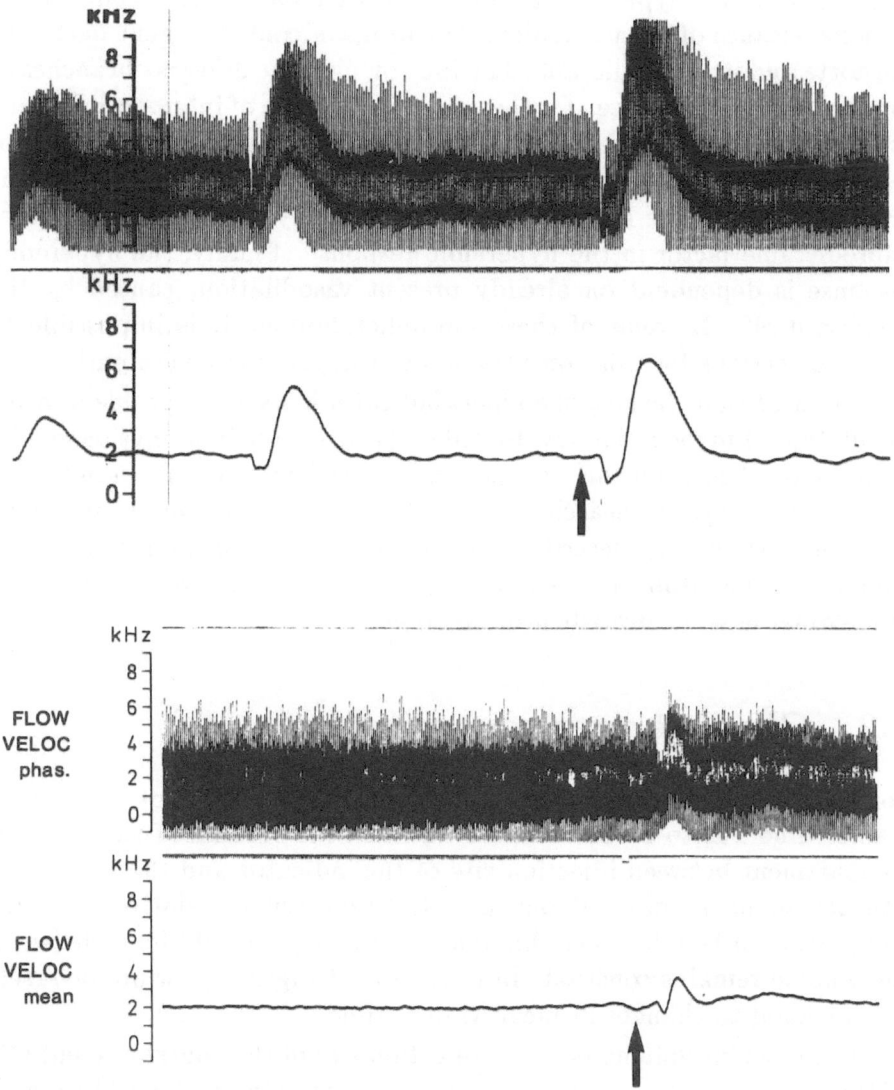

Figure 4.2: *Phasic and mean left circumflex artery flow after injection of 6 ml of the contrast agent diatrizoate (upper tracings) and after 6 ml of the low iodinate isoviscous and iso-osmolar contrast agent Iohexol-140 (lower tracings). Flow is represented by flow velocity and is expressed as the frequency shift of the Doppler signal, measured by an epicardial probe, which secures a constant diameter of the artery. The arrows indicate the moment of contrast injection.*

Moreover, the hyperemic response can vary for different contrast injections because of the unpredictable leakage of contrast agent back into the aorta and its unpredictable distribution over the different branches of the coronary arterial tree. Furthermore, in the case of interventions such as PTCA, higher flow through the dilated artery after a successful procedure will be accompanied by more of the contrast agent entering this branch than was the case before the angioplasty, constituting another unpredictable factor in the hyperemic response. Finally, the hyperemic response is dependent on already present vasodilation, caused by the stenosis itself. Because of these unpredictabilities, it is impossible to make corrections for this contrast induced hyperemia consistently.

It is clear that the lack of an inert indicator is a serious problem in the calculation of myocardial flow by videodensitometry in a physiologically sound way. The problems concerning contrast induced hyperemia and the in vain efforts to search for a contrast agent not influencing flow, are more extensively described in Appendix A. The final solution to circumvent this problem was found by restricting ourselves to the study of maximal flow, as described in Chapter 6.

4.2   Changes in vascular volume

For the calculation of flow according to equation 3.7, not only mean transit time has to be determined but also the volume of the vascular compartment between injection site of the indicator and the measuring site has to be known. If one is only interested in relative flow, i.e. comparison of flow between different situations, it would be sufficient if the volume remains constant. In that case, changes in flow are inversely proportional to changes in mean transit time.

The vascular volume between injection site of the contrast agent (tip of the coronary catheter) and its measuring site (the region of interest), however, does not remain constant at all: in the physiologic situation changes in coronary flow are induced by changes in arteriolar and capillary resistance and these, in turn, are caused by changes in vascular volume [6, 7, 8]. For this reason, calculation of coronary flow reserve by comparing time parameters alone, is precluded since the vascular volume is different in the resting and hyperemic state.

Clinical need is present to compare flow before and after interventions, such as PTCA or long-lasting lipid lowering therapy. If, however, the functional significance of a coronary artery stenosis has been changed by the intervention, this will result immediately in compensatory changes in peripheral resistance - and therefore volume - of the distal vascular bed, again precluding comparison of flow.

An approach which claimed to provide the solution of this problem was introduced by Vogel and coworkers several years ago [9, 10, 11, 12]. Vogel postulated that for every part of a myocardial region of interest, all blood in the corresponding vascular space would be totally replaced by contrast agent shortly after contrast injection. In that case measured density could be used as an index of volume. According to pathologic studies, however, the maximal volume of the vascular compartment of the heart is approximately 20 ml/100 g [13, 14, 15, 16], and while the vascular volume per unit increases from the left main coronary artery down to the capillary bed, the contrast bolus (6-8 ml) is actually dispersing. Therefore, it seems unlikely that undiluted contrast agent will pass through a myocardial region of interest at sites more distal to the injection site. The correctness of Vogel's postulate has been questioned for a long time and finally it could be proved that it is not true as will be shown in chapter 6.

A solution for the problem of the changing vascular volume was also found in the restriction to calculation of merely maximal flow as will be discussed later.

4.3 Contrast density vs contrast concentration

In the calculation of mean transit time from the concentration time curve $c(t)$ according to equation (3.11), concentration as a function of time should be known. What is measured in the catheterization laboratory, however, is the total amount of contrast density $d(t)$ in a layer perpendicular to the direction of the X-ray beams. Therefore, a large amount of density can either mean a large vascular compartment containing a low concentration of contrast agent or a smaller vascular compartment containing a higher contrast concentration (figure 4.3).

If, however, the vascular volume remains constant during image acquisition and between different situations in which flow is compared, one can state that density $d(t)$ is linearly proportional to concentration $c(t)$. Since in that case the numerator and denominator in equation 3.11 are both multiplied by the same factor, mean transit time can be calculated

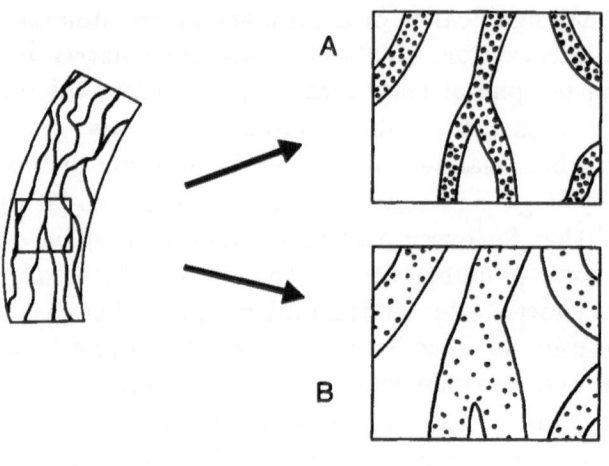

DENSITY ~ IODINE QUANTITY

~ IODINE CONCENTRATION

x

VASCULAR FRACTION

Figure 4.3: *Contrast density and contrast concentration are only directly proportional if the vascular volume remains constant.*

from the time-density curve instead of the virtual concentration-time curve.

To assure a linear relationship between $d(t)$ and $c(t)$, in fact a second condition has to been fulfilled: a linear relation should be present between the amount of iodine in a perpendicular section and the amount of density measured by the videochain. According to Lambert-Beer's law, attenuation of radiation is exponentially related to the amount of iodine in a perpendicular section. Therefore, pixel density values must be logarithmically transformed before subtraction. In chapter 5 it will be demonstrated that this can be fulfilled indeed in regular catheterization laboratory situations with net iodine layers not exceeding 0.5 cm (cf figure 5.3).

4.4   Difficulties in determination of mean transit time due to motion and insufficient image quality

Mean transit time of contrast passage through a certain part of the myocardium should be calculated from the time-density curve. This curve is obtained by sampling the average density within a region of interest at exactly identical moments in the heart cycle in a number of consecutive beats. The region of interest is chosen over the part of the myocardium which one wants to investigate. Because the heart is a moving object, the only way to ensure that the same region of interest is studied in every heart beat, is to avoid any kind of motion of the patient and to trigger the heart by atrial pacing at a constant rate, slightly above its own frequency. This means that images are taken, one per beat, at identical moments in the cardiac cycle. In our laboratory, triggering is performed just before onset of the QRS-complex when cardiac motion is relatively small. The last image before contrast injection (called the mask) is digitally subtracted from all the subsequent images which results in considerable enhancement of image quality and enables density analysis in myocardial regions of interest.

Such a motionless image acquisition is very demanding. In the first place, all evitable causes of motion, such as panning of the table, should be avoided. Next, the patient should be instructed not to move, which means that he should hold his breath carefully and should avoid any arbitrary motion of head, neck, shoulders and chest. Finally, special precautions should be taken in triggering as will be discussed below [17].

In clinical practice, image acquisition without marked motion artifacts has been tremendously difficult and most investigators did not succeed in obtaining an image quality enabling delineation of real indicator dilution curves [18, 19, 20]. Only the ascending part of the curve could be obtained reliably, corresponding with the first 5-7 beats after start of image acquisition. After the peak, the descending part of the curve did not return to the baseline again. Some authors have explained these slow kinetics of the washout phase by assuming extravasation of the contrast agent and even two-compartment models were postulated [18, 19, 20, 21, 22]. In chapter 6, however, it will be demonstrated that failure of the descending limb of the time-density curve to return to its baseline, is mostly due to insufficient image quality and other artifacts.

Because of these difficulties in determining mean transit time of contrast passage, a number of investigators have tried to substitute mean transit time by other time parameters earlier in the curve. Flow from one situation to another was compared by calculating ratios of these substituted parameters, such as appearance time, time of maximal inclination of the ascending limb, build up time, time of maximal contrast intensity, and many others [9], [10], [11], [18] - [24].

The most popular of these time parameters undoubtfully has been appearance time, defined in a different way by different authors but always referring to a moment somewhere in the first part of the curve (figure 6.4). Use of appearance time has the major advantage that this parameter is easily to obtain because only the ascending part of the curve has to be known, and that this moment mostly precedes the hyperemia induced by the contrast injection, a problem discussed earlier.

By implementing furthermore the postulate of Vogel about contrast density as an index of volume [9, 10, 11], flow could be represented by the ratio of maximal contrast intensity (D) and appearance time (T). Coronary flow reserve was determined by performing studies at baseline (b) and after a hyperemic stimulus (h) and expressed as:

$$\text{CFR} = \frac{D_h}{T_h} : \frac{D_b}{T_b} = \frac{D_h}{D_b} \times \frac{T_b}{T_h}$$

The results, obtained by this approach have been controversial. In the initial studies, reasonable correlations with measured flow were found but later studies have been disappointing [25]. Although this approach deserves the merit to have improved the familiarity of clinicians with ECG-triggered, digital radiography, *it should be emphasized that the substitution of mean transit time by other time parameters and the representation of vascular volume by maximal contrast intensity, are not supported by any physical or physiologic theory and are not correct as will be proved in chapter 6.*

It has always been our belief that it would be necessary to improve image quality and time-density curve quality in such a way that determination of mean transit time is possible in a reliable and reproducible way. This improvement has been achieved in a number of steps.

In the first place all patients are seen 24-48 hours before the planned catheterization at the outpatient's department. After explaining the aim of our efforts, thorough training to hold breath is performed at maximal inspiration during 20 seconds, using a nose clamp to prevent leakage of inspired air. Careful attention is paid to avoid any motion of head, neck, shoulders, chest and stomach. Thereafter, the patient is asked to exercise this holding of breath at home at night and also the next day after admission to the hospital. The catheterization itself is always performed by the same physician who gave the breathing instructions which promotes cooperation. In this way an excellent image quality is obtained in a large majority of patients.

The finishing touch in image quality is formed by using a special way of atrial stimulation, called *apparent cardiac arrest*. This method of triggering was introduced by Van der Werf in 1984 [17] and means that not only the heart itself is stimulated slightly above its inherent frequency, but also that synchrony exists between the X-ray pulses and the triggered heart beats. This is achieved by triggering the pacemaker as well as the X-ray generator by the divided videopulse [17].

Once the images and averaged densities within the myocardial regions of interest have been recorded, the sampled, discrete time-density curve is available. Thereafter, background regions of interest of identical size are chosen close to the myocardial regions of interest, but just outside the heart contour to detect changes in background density (cf figure 6.3 and figure 7.1). The average densities in the background are subtracted from the sampled data and a lognormal function or a gamma function is fitted to the remaining curve. By correction for changes in background density, a further increase in curve quality is usually obtained. More details about background correction and curve fitting will be described in chapter 6 and in appendix B.

4.5 Prerequisites for myocardial flow assessment by videodensitometry, according to the physiology of indicator dilution theory

From the former sections it can be concluded that evaluation of the value of videodensitometry for myocardial flow assessment, according to the principles of indicator dilution theory, would require:

1. *Images of such a high quality, that mean transit time can be determined unequivocally*

2. *A constant blood flow during image acquisition*

3. *A vascular volume which remains constant between different situations in which flow is compared.*

Only if these 3 conditions are fulfilled, flow from one situation to another will be inversely proportional to changes in mean transit time.

The first aim of our investigations was to test this theory in a flow model (chapter 5). Because in such a model the problems of influence of indicator on flow, changes in vascular volume and biological motion are not present, this study offered the possibilities to study the in-vitro value of the different parameters, to test fitting procedures and to test and calibrate densitometric calculations of our equipment.

The second step was to create an animal model in which all 3 conditions as mentioned above were fulfilled and to compare flow, as calculated by videodensitometry, and using mean transit time, with flow measured by a previously implanted flow probe (chapter 6).

The last step was to apply these results in man in a clinically feasible and useful way (chapter 7 and 8).

References

[1] Gerber K H and Higgins C B. Comparative effects of ionic and nonionic contrast materials on coronary and peripheral blood flow. *Invest Radiol*, 17:292–298, 1982.

[2] Schraeder R, Baller D, Hoeft A, Korb H, Wolpers H G, and Hellige G. Reduced side effects of low osmolality nonionic contrast media in coronary arteriography. In V Taenzer and E Zeitler, editors, *Contrast media in urography, angiography and computerized tomography*, pages 67–77. George Thieme Verlag, Stutgart, New York, 1983.

[3] Simon R, Koch M, Hermann G, Amende I, and Lichtlen P R. Direct effects of an ionic nonionic contrast agent on the coronary circulation in man. In *Proceedings Xth World Congress Cardiology*, page 294. Washington, 1986.

[4] Wilson R F, Laughlin D E, Ackell P H, Chilian W M, Holida M D, Hartley C J, Armstrong M L, Marcus M L, and White C W. Transluminal subselective measurement of coronary artery blood flow velocity and vasodilator reserve in man. *Circulation*, 72:82–92, 1985.

[5] Pijls N H J, Bos H S, Uijen G J H, and Van der Werf T. Is ionic isotonic iohexol the contrast agent of choice for quantitative myocardial videodensitometry? *Intern J Cardiac Imag*, 3:117–126, 1988.

[6] Gould K L, Lipscomb K, and Calvert C. Compensatory changes of the distal coronary vascular bed during progressive coronary constriction. *Circulation*, 51:1085–1094, 1975.

[7] Klopp E H and Gott V L. A simple model of the hemodynamic effects of a proximal coronary artery narrowing. *Ann Thorac Surg*, 19:309–312, 1975.

[8] White C W, Wright C B, Doty D B, Hiratza L F, Eastham C L, Harrison D G, and Marcus M L. Does visual interpretation of the coronary arteriogram predict the physiological importance of a coronary stenosis? *N Engl J Med*, 310:819–824, 1984.

[9] Hodgson J M, Legrand V, Bates E R, Mancini G B J, Aueron F M, O'Neill W W, Simon S B, Beauman G J, LeFree M T, and Vogel R A. Validation in dogs of a rapid digital angiographic technique to measure relative coronary blood flow during routine cardiac catheterization. *Am J Cardiol*, 55:188–193, 1985.

[10] Vogel R A. Radiographic assessment of coronary blood flow parameters. *Circulation*, 72:460–465, 1985.

[11] Bates E R, Aueron F M, Legrand V, LeFree M T, Mancini G B J, Hodgson J M, and Vogel R A. Comparative long-term effects of coronary artery bypass graft surgery and percutaneous transluminal coronary angioplasty on regional coronary flow reserve. *Circulation*, 72:833–839, 1985.

[12] Cusma J T, Toggart E J, Folts J D, Peppler W W, Hagiandreou N J, Lee C S, and Mistretta C A. Digital subtraction imaging of coronary flow reserve. *Circulation*, 75:461–472, 1987.

[13] Crystal G J, Downey H F, and Bashour F A. Small vessel and total coronary blood volume during intracoronary adenosine. *Am J Physiol*, 241:H194–H201, 1981.

[14] Weiss H R and Winbury M M. Nitroglycerine and chromonar on small-vessel content of the ventricular walls. *Am J Physiol*, 226:838–843, 1974.

[15] O'Keefe D D, Hoffman J I E, Cheitlin R, O'Neill M J, Allard J R, and Shapkin E. Coronary blood flow in experimental canine left ventricular hyperthrophy. *Circ Res*, 43:43–51, 1978.

[16] Bassingthwaighte J B, Yipinstoi T, and Harvey R B. Microvasculature of the dog left ventricular myocardium. *Microvasc Res*, 7:229–249, 1974.

[17] Van der Werf T, Heethaar R M, Stegehuis H, and Meijler F L. The concept of apparent cardiac arrest as a prerequisite for coronary digital subtraction angiography. *J Am Coll Cardiol*, 4:239–244, 1984.

[18] Nishimura R A, Rogers P J, Holmes D R, Gehring D G, and Bove A A. Assessment of myocardial perfusion by videodensitometry in the canine model. *J Am Coll Cardiol*, 9:891–897, 1987.

[19] Toggart E J and Mistretta C A. Digital coronary angiography: approaches using intravenous and direct methods. In G B J Mancini, editor, *Clinical applications of cardiac digital angiography*, pages 253–279. Raven Press, New York, 1988.

[20] Vogel R A and Mancini G B J. Assessment of coronary flow and myocardial perfusion with digital radiography. In G B J Mancini, editor, *Clinical applications of cardiac digital angiography*, pages 281–290. Raven Press, New York, 1988.

[21] Spiller P, Schmiel F K, Politz B, Block M, Fermor U, Hackbarth W, Jehle J, Korfer R, and Pannek H. Measurement of systolic and diastolic flow rates in the coronary artery system by x-ray videodensitometry. *Circulation*, 68:337–347, 1983.

[22] Nissen S E, Elion J L, Booth D C, Evans J, and DeMaria A N. Value and limitations of computer analysis of digital subtraction angiography in the assessment of coronary flow reserve. *Circulation*, 73:562–571, 1986.

[23] Zijlstra F, Reiber J C, Juilliere Y, and Serruys P W. Normalizaiton of coronary flow reserve by percutaneous transluminal coronary angioplasty. *Am J Cardiol*, 61:55–60, 1988.

[24] Serruys P W, Juilliere Y, Zijlstra F, Beatt K J, De Feyter P J, Suryapranata H, Van den Brand M, and Roelandt J. Coronary blood flow velocity during percutaneous transluminal coronary angioplasty as a guide for assessment of the functional result. *Am J Cardiol*, 61:253–259, 1988.

[25] Hess O M, McGillem M, DeBoe S F, Pinto I M F, Callegher K P, and Mancini G B J. Determination of coronary flow reserve by parametric imaging. *Circulation*, 82:1438–1448, 1990.

Replacement of page 51

Replacement of page 52

Chapter 5

A Model Study to Validate Calculation of Myocardial Blood Flow by Videodensitometry

5.1 Introduction

From the principles of indicator dilution theory it is known that after injection of an indicator into a steady state flow system, flow can be calculated from the dilution curve by the ratio of vascular volume between injection site and sampling site and mean transit time [1]. In a one compartment model, the indicator dilution curve consists of a short rapid upstroke, followed by a monoexponential decline representing the wash-out phase [1].

Mean transit time (T_{mn}) is defined as the average time, needed by a particle of indicator to travel from injection site to measuring site and, as outlined in chapter 3, can be derived by the dilution curve c(t) by the equation:

$$T_{mn} = \frac{\int_0^\infty t \cdot c(t) \cdot dt}{\int_0^\infty c(t) \cdot dt} \tag{5.1}$$

Injection of contrast agent into a coronary artery as routinely performed during cardiac catheterization, is followed by opacification of the myocardium supplied by that particular artery and subsequent wash-out. After introduction of the principles of digital subtraction imaging and apparent cardiac arrest in coronary arteriography (cf section 3.3 and 4.4), it has been become possible to visualize this passage of contrast agent through the myocardium and to obtain time-density curves

53

by videodensitometry [2, 3, 4, 5]. These time-density curves resemble dye dilution curves, and many investigators tried to predict coronary and myocardial blood flow from different time parameters derived from these curves [6, 7, 8, 9, 10].

These time-density curves, however, cannot strictly be treated as indicator dilution curves because of several reasons. Besides the problems listed in chapter 4, which are inherent to living beings, there are two more points which have to be solved beforehand. In the first place, the amount of injected contrast agent is not negligibly small and therefore influences flow. In the second place, a prerequisite to derive mean transit time from the dilution curve is linearity of the Y-axis, i.e. existence of a linear relationship between the amount of contrast agent (# of iodine particles) in a myocardial region of interest (ROI) and the density value attributed to this ROI [1]. In fact this means that Lambert-Beer's law should be applicable in the appropriate range of densities, which is not obvious because usual X-ray radiation is not monochromatic. Therefore, after logarithmical transformation of assigned density, a linear relation between the amount of iodine in a perpendicular section and the density value assigned to that section has to be verified empirically before calculation of mean transit time can be performed. One aim of this study was therefore to investigate if Lambert-Beer's law can be reliably applied to situations as encountered in a regular digital catheterization laboratory.

As outlined in section 4.4, a number of time parameters different from T_{mn} have been used to predict flow ratios [4, 6, 7, 8, 11, 12, 13, 14]. Use of these other parameters is not supported by any physical or physiologic theory. For this reason, their respective suitability to replace T_{mn} should be tested in a flow model in which flow and vascular volume can be completely controlled. The second aim of this study was therefore to examine the accuracy of these substituted time parameters to predict relative flow in such a hydrodynamic flow model, not susceptible to biological variations. Because the vascular volume of this model was exactly known, the additional advantage was offered to investigate what is the best possible approximation of absolute flow by videodensitometry under ideal circumstances, using regular catheterization laboratory equipment.

In clinical situations the time-density curve is a sampled curve, consisting of a limited number of discrete data. For calculation of T_{mn} from this curve, extrapolation and adequate curve fitting are mandatory. These are mathematical problems which obviously can be studied best in a model circulation. Investigation of procedures for extrapolation and curve fitting for this application was a further aim of this study.

5.2 Materials and methods

5.2.1 Flow model

The flow model in this study consisted of silastic tube (inner diameter 4.0 mm) simulating the coronary arteries and an especially constructed system of 10000 parallel running polypropylene capillaries (inner diameter $10\mu m$, Asahi Medical Co., Tokyo) simulating the myocardial capillary bed (figure 5.1). Because theoretically mean transit time and flow are inversely proportional provided that vascular volume remains constant, and because the maximum acquisition time of our digital X-ray equipment is 20 seconds in the ECG-triggered mode at an acquisition rate of 2 frames/s, it was necessary to use capillary beds corresponding with 3 different vascular volumes (7, 17 and 41 ml respectively) to provide the opportunity for flow measurement over a wide range of 6 to 300 ml/min. Low flow rates were defined in this study as 6-48 ml/min in steps of 6 ml/min, medium flow rates as 60-96 ml/min in steps of 12 ml/min and high flow rates as 100-300 ml/min in steps of 25 ml/min. The model was perfused by NaCl 0.9%. Flow was generated by a roller pump (Watson-Marlow MHRE Flow Inducer) and measured by an electromagnetic flow meter (Skalar Transflow 601). Inherent pulsations of the roller pump were damped by an air chamber. The flow meter was calibrated by measuring the filling time of a graduated cylinder and this calibration was repeated before each contrast injection.

5.2.2 Image acquisition and processing

A 5F NIH catheter was advanced into the tubular system through an Y-connector (ACS 23242). Contrast injections of 1, 2 and 2 ml iohexol-140 respectively were performed using an angiographic power injector (Sybron Angiomat 300) with an injection rate of 2, 4 and 4 ml/s for the low, medium and high flow rates, respectively. Contrast injection started automatically 2.5 s after the start of image acquisition to provide a stable baseline (zero density level). The moment at which half of the contrast bolus was injected, was defined as $t = 0$. The background for the model consisted of a 10 cm layer of perspex simulating human tissues, and a 1

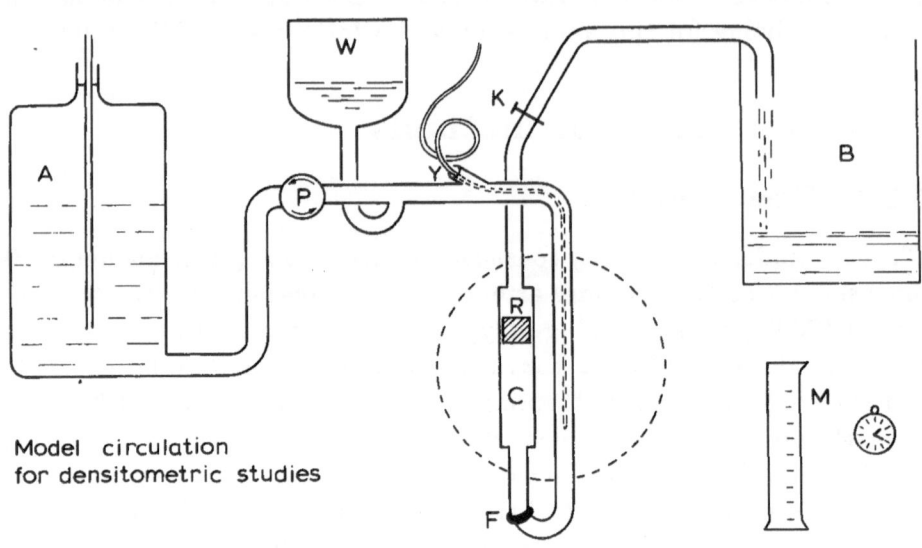

Figure 5.1: *Model circulation used in this study. A: Afferent reservoir, D: Roller Pump, W: Air Chamber, Y: Y-connector for introduction of catheter, F: Electromagnetic flow meter, C: Capillary bed, R: Region of Interest over the capillary bed, K: Resistance Clamp, B: Efferent reservoir, M: Graduated cylinder and stopwatch for calibration of the EM flow meter. The dotted circle indicates the position of the image intensifier.*

mm Al filter as required by Health Authorities to eliminate low-energetic radiation [15].

Image acquisition and processing were performed using a Siemens Bicor X-ray equipment in connection with a Siemens Digitron 3 computer for digital subtraction angiography. Image acquisition was performed using a fixed kilovoltage and a fixed milliamperage (100 mA) at an acquisition rate of 2 frames/s during 20 s. Regions of interest (ROIs) were chosen close to the tip of the coronary catheter to record onset of contrast injection and over the central part of the capillary bed. For study of the fitting procedures, a number of other ROIs were chosen over the afferent tube and the capillary bed. Close to all ROIs, background ROIs were chosen of identical size, just outside the model, to detect changes in background density. After logarithmic amplification, images were digi-

tized in 512×512 matrices with 1024 density levels, with a 10 bits ADC
at a rate of 22 MHz and stored subsequently.

5.2.3 Absorption characteristics

To examine the applicability of Lambert-Beer's law for contrast layers
as used in this study, a calibration block was constructed consisting of
8 cubes with an edge of 1 cm filled with different dilutions of regular
diatrizoate (Urographin-370) in saline (1/2, 1/4, 1/8, 1/16, 1/32, 1/64,
1/128 and 0). The iodine content of these cubes corresponded with pure
diatrizoate layers with a thickness between 0 and 0.5 cm or iohexol-140
layers between 0 and 1.3 cm. Image acquisition of the calibration block
was performed during 10 seconds with a rate of 2 frames/s and with a
background as described above. This was repeated after addition to the
background of 4 different Cu-filters with a thickness of 0.5, 1.0, 1.5 and
2.0 mm respectively to absorb high energetic radiation and to obtain
an additional narrowing of the radiation spectrum. The respective kilo-
voltages in this part of the study were 63 without Cu-filter and 66, 77,
85 and 90 kV for the respective Cu-filters. To prevent cancellation of
the calibration block by the subtraction procedure, this block was connected to a pneumatic piston to enable movement of the block during
image acquisition (figure 5.2). For analysis of density calculation, ROIs
of 15×15 pixels were chosen over every cube and over its corresponding
background.

5.2.4 Processing of time-density curves

The sequence of averaged pixel densities in a region of interest in the
images representing the consecutive heart cycles can be considered as a
sampled contrast dilution curve, the time density curve d(t). In practice this curve is superposed upon a background density. Background
level and curve parameters can be obtained in one operation by using
a general fitting procedure on the sampled data. Several mathematical
functions can be used and from these we have tested the lognormal function and the gamma function. Details about these fits are described in
Appendix B. The quality of the fits was judged by calculating the relative error between the sampled data and the fit. If the fit was considered
to be representative for the sampled data, the different time parameters
were calculated as follows: appearance time (T_{app}) was defined as the

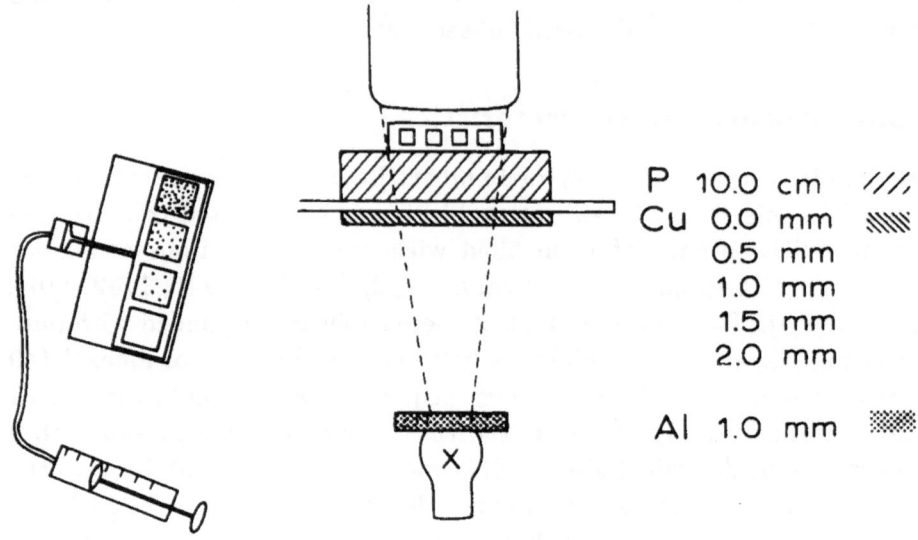

P   10.0 cm   ///
Cu   0.0 mm   \\\\
      0.5 mm
      1.0 mm
      1.5 mm
      2.0 mm

Al   1.0 mm   ▓▓

Figure 5.2: *Calibration block as used in this study to verify applicability of Lambert-Beer's law, and position of the block and the different filters. Al = Aluminium, I = image intensifier, C = calibration block, Cu = Copper, P = perspex, X = X-ray tube.*

time at which the fit function exceeded a value of 1% of the maximal contrast intensity, time of maximal contrast intensity (T_{max}) as the time corresponding with the top of the fitted curve, build up time (T_{bu}) as the difference of T_{max} and T_{app}, while T_{mn} was calculated from the fit according to theory, using equation (5.1).

5.2.5   Relation between flow and time parameters

The relation between flow and the inverse values of the different time parameters was evaluated by calculation of separate correlation coefficients for the low, medium and high flow rates using the least square regression method. For the calculation of absolute flow by videodensitometry, the vascular volume V between the tip of the catheter and the center of the regarding region of interest was calculated by adding the volumetrically determined content of the tubular part of the model and the content of the concerning part of the capillary bed as provided by the manufacturer. Densitometric flow F was defined as V/T_{mn} and compared with electromagnetic flow for all flow rates.

5.3 Results

5.3.1 Applicability of Lambert-Beer's law

For the evaluation of linearity between the amount of contrast agent in a perpendicular section and the assigned density value on an arbitrary scale from 0 to 1023, the average pixel densities for the concerning ROIs were computed (table 5.1). After background correction the relation between average density and Iodine content of the eight cubes was studied for the different Cu-filters (figure 5.3). For practical reasons these results are plotted on a logarithmic scale. For all Cu- filters used as well as for the situation without Cu-filter the relation is almost linear and the correlation coefficients are close to 1.00.

5.3.2 Fitting of the curves

An adequate fit could always be obtained by both fitting procedures, using all sampled data between 0 and the time at which the density in the wash-out phase became less than 60% of the maximal density. The relative error Er was always less than 10% for the time-density curves, obtained from the capillary ROIs. The average Er was slightly smaller for the lognormal fit than was the case for the gammafit. Reproducibility of T_{mn}, determined from 9 consecutive contrast injections at the same flow rate for 4 different capillary ROIs, was slightly better for the gamma function. More details about curve fitting are described in appendix B. Some representative examples of a background corrected time-density curves and the corresponding lognormal fits are presented in figure 5.4.

5.3.3 Assessment of relative flow

The relations between inverse time parameters and electromagnetic flow are summarized in table 5.2 for all four time parameters and for the low, medium and high flow rates. For flow rates between 50 and 300 ml/min a good correlation exists using all time parameters. For flow rates less than 50 ml/min, the inverse values of maximum concentration time, build up time and mean transit time still show a good correlation with electromagnetic flow. For appearance time, however, no correlation is present anymore.

Table 5.1: *Average pixel density in the ROIs over the calibration block (R) and in the corresponding background ROIs (B) on a scale of 0-1023 units as well as the differences (R-B). The results are presented without and with the different copper filters. ROIs are indicated by the U-370 dilution in the corresponding cube.*

ROI	0.0 mm CU			0.5 mm CU		
$2^{-n} \times U370$	R	B	R-B	R	B	R-B
n = 1	940.4	328.5	611.9	821.9	293.1	528.8
n = 2	680.7	322.6	358.1	567.1	287.8	288.3
n = 3	503.2	314.7	188.5	430.4	282.1	148.3
n = 4	406.0	309.0	97.0	351.3	274.0	77.3
n = 5	369.3	321.2	48.1	322.5	284.0	38.5
n = 6	345.7	318.9	26.6	304.4	283.7	20.7
n = 7	335.5	319.1	16.1	295.8	283.9	11.9
n = ∞	329.4	318.3	11.1	290.8	282.9	7.9

ROI	1.0 mm CU			1.5 mm CU		
$2^{-n} \times U370$	R	B	R-B	R	B	R-B
n = 1	650.2	339.3	310.9	467.0	219.3	247.7
n = 2	510.1	335.4	174.7	339.2	215.1	124.1
n = 3	424.2	330.6	93.6	285.7	211.8	73.9
n = 4	373.7	323.5	50.2	249.7	206.5	43.2
n = 5	354.7	336.6	21.1	240.3	219.6	20.7
n = 6	342.0	330.8	11.2	230.5	218.4	12.1
n = 7	335.7	228.5	7.2	227.8	220.0	7.8
n = ∞	335.8	332.6	3.2	226.5	223.4	3.1

ROI	2.0 mm CU		
$2^{-n} \times U370$	R	B	R-B
n = 1	328.9	180.4	148.5
n = 2	254.2	177.1	77.1
n = 3	212.8	173.5	39.3
n = 4	190.0	169.8	20.2
n = 5	189.9	179.9	10.0
n = 6	183.9	176.7	6.2
n = 7	181.3	176.4	4.7
n = ∞	180.8	177.9	2.9

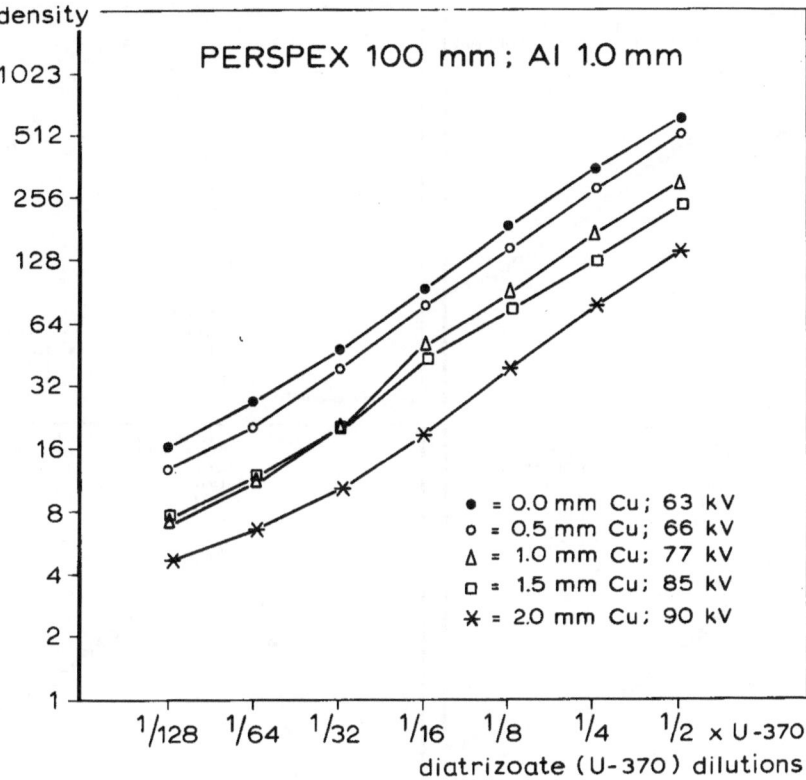

Figure 5.3: *Relation between different dilutions of U-370 in saline in a one centimeter perpendicular section and assigned density value on a scale of 0-1023 arbitrary density units (bilogarithmic scale).*

5.3.4 Assessment of absolute flow

For every flow rate, absolute flow was calculated densitometrically by dividing vascular volume between injection site and the center of the ROI over the capillary bed and mean transit time derived from the time-density curve d(t), according to equation (5.1) by substitution of $d(t)$ for $c(t)$. This substitution is permitted because the volume of the model was constant. The comparison of densitometrically computed flow and measured electromagnetic flow is presented in figure 5.5. For flow rates higher than 25 ml/min, densitometric flow approximates electromagnetic flow very well. The absolute value of the percentual difference

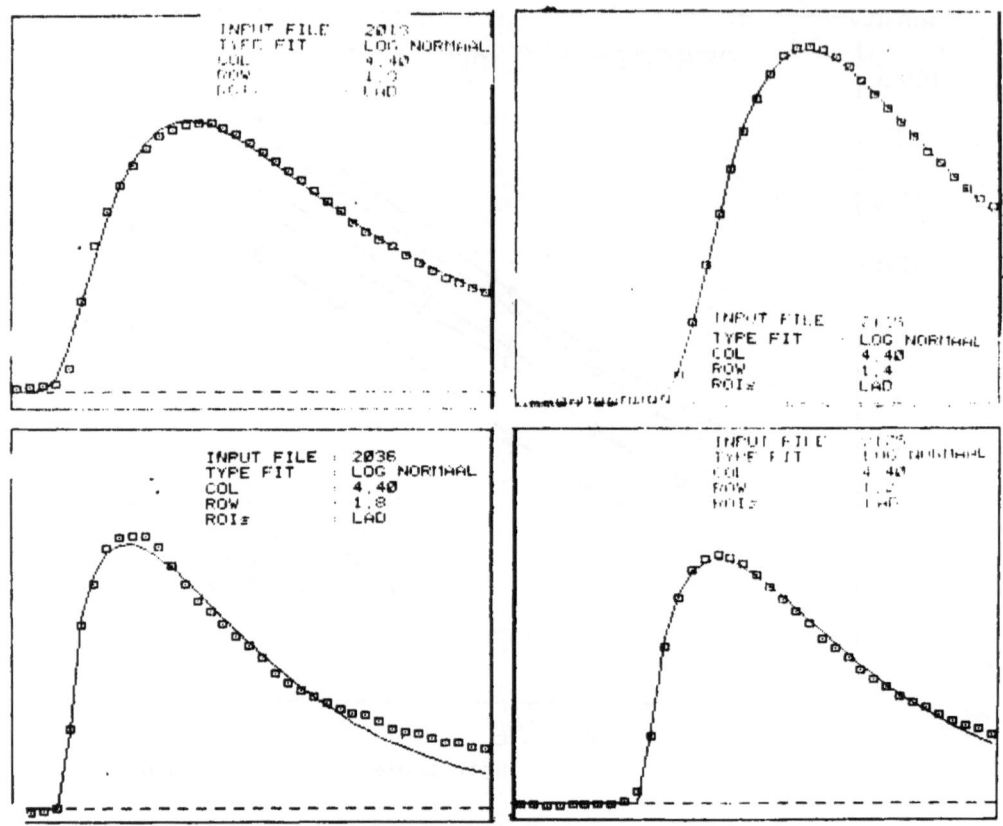

Figure 5.4: *Some examples of background corrected time density curves (squares) and their lognormal fits (dotted lines) corresponding with flow rates of 18 ml/min (upper left), 36 ml/min (lower left), 125 ml/min (upper right) and 175 ml/min (lower right).*

between both values was $7.3 \pm 6.4\%$ in this range. At flow rates of less than 25 ml/min, however, progressive overestimation of flow by the densitometric computation occurs.

5.4 Discussion

In this hydrodynamic flow model we tried to approximate the ideal situation of indicator dilution theory as well as possible, using regular catheterization laboratory equipment and using contrast agent as the in-

Table 5.2: *Correlation coefficients between inverse time parameters and flow, as well as the interception with the Y-axis.*

corr. coeff.	$1/T_{app}$	$1/T_{bu}$	$1/T_{mn}$	$1/T_{max}$
low flow	-0.21	0.96	0.96	0.98
medium flow	0.86	0.98	0.93	0.99
high flow	0.98	0.89	0.97	0.95
interception (s^{-1})	$1/T_{app}$	$1/T_{bu}$	$1/T_{mn}$	$1/T_{max}$
low flow	-2.40	0.06	0.09	0.06
medium flow	0.20	-0.25	-0.17	0.08
high flow	0.04	-0.07	-0.03	-0.04

dicator. Almost instantaneous injection of contrast agent was performed at the origin of a single compartment system in a dynamic equilibrium. Changes in this equilibrium due to biological variability were excluded and the vascular volume of the model was exactly known. Nevertheless, the amount of contrast agent used in this study was still not negligible compared to flow. Use of lower amounts of contrast agents, however, is not realistic. From animal and clinical studies we know that this quantity of a low iodinated contrast agent is the absolute minimum to obtain subtraction images of a reasonable quality [13].

This study was performed using flow rates between 6 and 300 ml/min which represent the range of coronary flow in large dogs and humans [16, 17, 18, 19]. A shortcoming we had not realized beforehand, was that no leakage of redundant indicator was possible as is the case in animal and man. Another difference with a real vascular bed is that in our model all branching occurred at the entrance and that all capillaries were running parallel without intersections.

We investigated if Lambert-Beer's law can be assumed to be applicable using our catheterization laboratory equipment and using contrast layers up to 0.5 cm of a regular contrast agent (370 mg I/ml) or up to 1.3 cm of a low iodinated agent (140 mg I/ml). Even if taking into account that overprojection of different parts of myocardium occurs during coronary arteriography, it is unlikely that the total thickness of the underlying vascular compartment will exceed these values [20]. In all studies we ever performed the highest density values after coronary contrast injec-

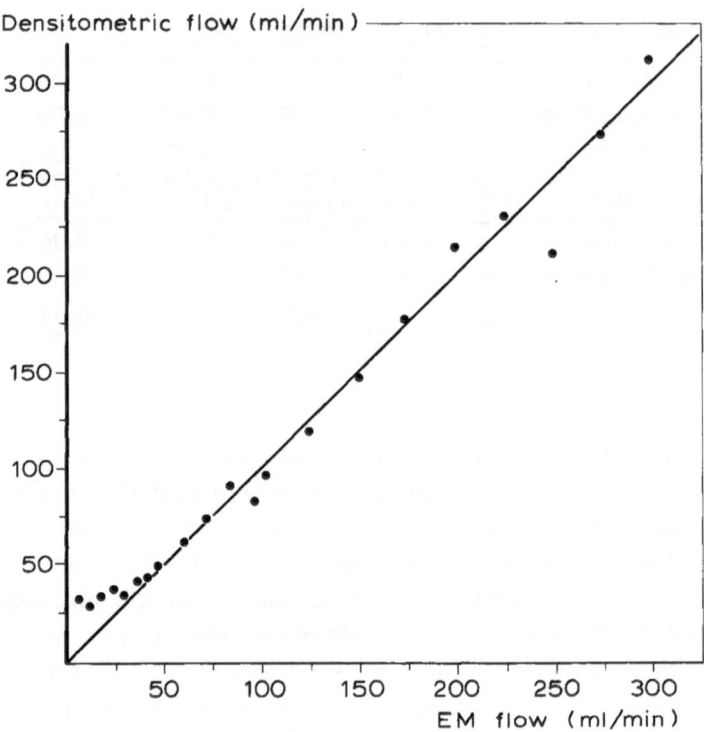

Figure 5.5: *Relation between flow measured by the electromagnetic flow meter and flow calculated by videodensitometry. The line indicates the line of identity.*

tion were attributed to the proximal parts of the large coronary arteries themselves and even if blood would be completely replaced by contrast agent, this layer thickness will not exceed 5 mm. Therefore, linearity between amount of contrast agent in a perpendicular layer and density value assigned by the Digitron, can be assumed.

Time parameters in this study were derived from the time- density curve $d(t)$. Because of the linearity demonstrated above and because of the constant vascular volume in this study, substitution of $d(t)$ for the dilution curve $c(t)$ is justified as far as calculation of time parameters is concerned: numerator and denominator in equation (5.1) are multiplied by the same constant value.

In the assessment of flow ratios by ratios of time parameters, mean transit time and maximal concentration time provided good results. Appearance time, however, became increasingly less accurate for lower flow rates. In fact, from this model study and also from later animal studies, we learned that the closer a certain time parameter to T_{mn}, the better its adequacy to assess flow correctly.

Except for the fact that these results are in accordance with theory, some other points may have contributed to the poor results obtained in this study when using T_{app}. In the first place it should be remarked that the vascular volume at low and medium flow rates was considerably less than at high flow rates (7, 17 and 41 ml respectively) whereas the amount of contrast agent (1, 2 and 2 ml respectively) in relation to flow was substantially higher at the lower flow rates. Appearance time is obviously most sensitive for this relation between vascular volume, injected volume and injection rate. Another factor possibly contributing to the inaccuracy of appearance time is the inappropriate temporal resolution at an image acquisition rate of 2 frames/s, which is relatively worse for appearance time than for the other time parameters defined later in the curve. This rather poor temporal resolution could have been improved by a faster acquisition rate. This would have resulted, however, in a shorter time available for acquisition because the maximal number of images which can be obtained in one session is 40 in the ECG-triggered mode of our equipment. A shorter acquisition time would have resulted in premature break-off of the time-density curves. Moreover, in the living being in which one image per heart cycle has to be obtained, faster rates than 2/s will not be used.

Because flow rates below 50 ml/min are quite often encountered in the human coronary bed [16, 17, 18, 19], the results of this study, notwithstanding its inherent shortcomings, seem to warn to fallacious results of flow assessment by appearance time alone in patients with important coronary artery stenosis.

In this study densitometric flow could be calculated from the vascular volume and mean transit time. A fairly good correlation with electromagnetic flow was found at flow rates higher than 25 ml/min. At lower flow rates, however, progressive overestimation of flow by densitometric calculation occurred. This may also be explained by the volume and injection rate of the injected contrast bolus (1 ml in 0.5 s) in comparison with the vascular volume (7 ml). This represents a considerable flow disturbance at these low flow rates and thus violates the steady flow assumption. As mentioned earlier, in the animal or catheterization laboratory this last problem will be less important because the excess of injected indicator can leak away into the aorta and no more contrast agent will enter the coronary circulation as permitted by instantaneous coronary flow.

Attempting to extrapolate the results of this study to animal or human studies, it is unlikely that in vivo estimation of myocardial flow by densitometry can be better than the results of this model study and it can be expected that similar good results can only be obtained if biological variations during acquisition of the time-density curve or between different studies are minimized. Changes in vascular volume or flow during acquisition of the curve have to be avoided. As will be shown in the next chapters, this can be reached by induction of maximal hyperemia during the study by i.v. administration of dipyridamole or by i.c. administration of papaverine prior to contrast injection.

5.5   Conclusions

From this model study it can be concluded that densitometrically determined flow correlates well with electromagnetic flow measurement, provided that the vascular volume does not change and flow itself remains constant during image acquisition.

Of the four time parameters analyzed in this study, T_{mn} and T_{max} showed the best inverse relation with flow. Using T_{app}, a reliable result was only obtained at flow rates higher than 50 ml/min.

Therefore, at lower flow rates, as often encountered in clinical situations, where even resting flow may be jeopardized by a severe coronary stenosis, use of the physiologic time parameter T_{mn} to assess flow ratios is advisable if at least reliable determination of this time parameter is permitted by adequate image and time-density curve quality. Feasibility of such an image quality will be demonstrated in chapter 7.

References

[1] Zierler K L. *Circulation times and the theory of indicator dilution methods for determining blood flow and volume*, pages 585–615. American Physiological Society, Washington DC, 1962.

[2] Rutishauser W, Simon H, Stucky J P, Schad N, Noseda G, and Wellauer J. Evaluation of roentgen cinedensitometry for flow measurement in models and in the intact circulation. *Circulation*, 36:951–963, 1967.

[3] Smith H C, Frye R I, Donald D E, Davis G D, Pluth J R, Sturm R E, and Wood E H. Roentgen videodensitometric measurement of coronary blood flow. determination from simultaneous indicator-dilution curves at selected sites in the coronary circulation and in coronary artery-saphenous vein grafts. *Mayo Clin Proc*, 46:800–806, 1971.

[4] Vogel R A, Bates E R, O'Neill W W, Aueron F M, Meier B, and Gruentzig A R. Coronary flow reserve measured during cardiac catheterization. *Arch Intern Med*, 144:1773–1776, 1984.

[5] Van der Werf T, Heethaar R M, Stegehuis H, and Meijler F L. The concept of apparent cardiac arrest as a prerequisite for coronary digital subtraction angiography. *J Am Coll Cardiol*, 4:239–244, 1984.

[6] Vogel R, LeFree M, Bates E, O'Neill W, Foster R, Kirlin P, Smith D, and Pitt B. Application of digital techniques to selective coronary arteriography: use of myocardial appearance time to measure coronary flow reserve. *Am Heart J*, 107:153–164, 1984.

[7] Bates E R, Aueron F M, Legrand V, LeFree M T, Mancini G B J, Hodgson J M, and Vogel R A. Comparative long-term effects of coronary artery bypass graft surgery and percutaneous transluminal coronary angioplasty on regional coronary flow reserve. *Circulation*, 72:833–839, 1985.

[8] Cusma J T, Toggart E J, Folts J D, Peppler W W, Hagiandreou N J, Lee C S, and Mistretta C A. Digital subtraction imaging of coronary flow reserve. *Circulation*, 75:461–472, 1987.

[9] Van der Werf T, Heethaar R M, Stegehuis H, Pijls N H J, and Meijler F L. *Comparison of time parameters derived from myocardial time-density curves in patients before and after percutaneous transluminal coronary angioplasty*, pages 227–236. Martinus Nijhoff, Dordrecht, Lancaster, Boston, 1988.

[10] Ikeda H, Koga Y, Utsu F, and Toshima H. Quantitative evaluation of regional myocardial blood flow by videodensitometric analysis of digital subtraction coronary arteriography in humans. *J Am Coll Cardiol*, 8:809–816, 1986.

[11] Gerber K H and Higgins C B. Comparative effects of ionic and nonionic contrast materials on coronary and peripheral blood flow. *Invest Radiol*, 17:292–298, 1982.

[12] Hodgson J M B, Mancini G B J, Legrand V, and Vogel R A. Characterization of changes in coronary blood flow during the first six seconds after intracoronary contrast injection. *Invest Radiol*, 20:246–252, 1985.

[13] Pijls N H J, Bos H S, Uijen G J H, and Van der Werf T. Is ionic isotonic iohexol the contrast agent of choice for quantitative myocardial videodensitometry? *Intern J Cardiac Imag*, 3:117–126, 1988.

[14] Zijlstra F, Reiber J C, Juilliere Y, and Serruys P W. Normalizaiton of coronary flow reserve by percutaneous transluminal coronary angioplasty. *Am J Cardiol*, 61:55–60, 1988.

[15] Curry T S, Dowdey J E, and Murry R C. *Christensen's introduction to the physics of diagnostic radiology*, pages 77–81. Philadelphia, 1984.

[16] Rubio R and Berne R M. Regulation of coronary blood flow. *Progress in cardiovascular diseases*, 18:105–122, 1975.

[17] Vatner S F, Higgins C B, and Braunwald E. Effects of norepinephrine on coronary circulation and left ventricular dynamics in the conscious dog. *Circ Res*, 34:812–823, 1974.

[18] Gould K L, Lipscomb K, and Calvert C. Compensatory changes of the distal coronary vascular bed during progressive coronary constriction. *Circulation*, 51:1085–1094, 1975.

[19] Marcus M L. Labeled microspheres. In M L Marcus, editor, *The coronary circulation in health and disease*, pages 34–38. McGraw-Hill, New York, 1983.

[20] Piek J J and Becker A E. Collateral blood supply to the myocardium at risk in human myocardial infarction: a quantitative postmortem study. *J Am Coll Cardiol*, 11:1290–1296, 1988.

Replacement of page 69

Replacement of page 70

Chapter 6

Mean Transit Time for the Assessment of Myocardial Perfusion by Videodensitometry

6.1 Introduction

Early studies about calculation of coronary blood flow by analysis of contrast agent passage in the coronary arteriogram were reported more than 2 decades ago by Rutishauser et al. and Smith et al [1, 2, 3, 4]. Shortly thereafter, it was shown that visualization of contrast passage through the myocardium could be enhanced by ECG-triggered digital subtraction imaging [5] and it was suggested that myocardial flow could be calculated by studying the temporal changes in contrast intensity in a myocardial region of interest (ROI) as a function of time: the time-density curve (TDC). According to the principles of indicator dilution theory [6], outlined in more detail in chapter 3, flow (F) can be calculated from these TDCs by the equation:

$$F = V/T_{mn} \qquad (6.1)$$

where V represents the volume of the vascular bed between the injection site of the contrast agent (i.e. the tip of the coronary catheter) and the measuring site, and where T_{mn} represents the mean transit time of the contrast particles. T_{mn} is calculated from the time-density curve $d(t)$ according to the equation:

$$T_{mn} = \frac{\int_0^\infty t \cdot d(t) \cdot dt}{\int_0^\infty d(t) \cdot dt} \qquad (6.2)$$

In vivo calculation of flow in this way however, is complicated by a number of problems, which are discussed extensively in chapter 4. The most important problems are: 1. Flow F is not constant during the acquisition of the TDC because of the hyperemic response to the contrast injection [7, 8], 2. the vascular volume V is unknown and not constant from one situation to another, and 3. accurate computation of T_{mn} requires high quality image acquisition without motion artifacts during approximately 15-20 heart beats.

As extensively discussed in chapter 4, several solutions for these problems have been suggested. Current approaches are commonly derived in one or the other way from the method introduced by Vogel and coworkers and are based on two major assumptions [9, 10, 11, 12, 13, 14]: The mean transit time T_{mn} in equation (6.1) is generally replaced by some other time parameter of which contrast appearance time (T_{app}) is the most popular [9, 10, 12, 13, 15, 16]. This time parameter precedes the hyperemic response to contrast agent and has the additional advantage that only the first part of the TDC has to be obtained to determine this time parameter. Other time parameters have also been used to replace mean transit time [2, 16, 17, 18, 19, 20, 21]. Additionally, it is hypothetized that vascular volume V can be represented by the ROI-averaged maximal contrast intensity, assuming that all blood in the vascular compartment will be completely replaced by contrast agent at some moment during contrast passage [12, 14, 19].

This approach has empirically proved to be useful in animal and human studies and has considerably contributed to the introduction of flow assessment by videodensitometry in clinical practice [12, 13, 15],[22] - [25]. Nevertheless it should be emphasized that neither the use of T_{app} instead of T_{mn} nor representation of vascular volume by maximal contrast intensity is supported by any physical or physiologic theory. Investigation of the value of videodensitometry for myocardial flow assessment according to the original physiologic principles would require improvement of image quality to enable determination of T_{mn} from the TDC in an unequivocal and reproducible way, constant blood flow during the acquisition of the TDC itself, and a vascular volume which remains constant between different situations in which flow is compared. If all these conditions are fullfilled, flow from one situation to another is inversely proportional to T_{mn}, according to equation (6.1).

The aims of this study in dogs were therefore 1. to achieve such an improvement of image and TDC quality, 2. to investigate the feasibility of T_{mn} for the assessment of myocardial perfusion using a dog model in which vascular volume was kept constant and flow was not influenced by contrast injection and 3. to analyze the validity of the two major assumptions as described above about replacement of T_{mn} by other time parameters and representation of vascular volume by maximal contrast intensity.

6.2 Methods

6.2.1 Animal instrumentation and experimental protocol

After premedication with 0.1 mg fentanyl, 5.0 mg droperidol and 0.5 mg atropine i.m., 8 mongrel dogs of either sex (average weight 32 kg, range 26 - 36 kg) were anesthetized with sodium pentobarbital 25 mg/kg i.v. and ventilated by room air/ethrane. Under sterile conditions a left thoracotomy was performed, the pericardium was opened and epicardial pacing electrodes were sutured on the left atrium. The proximal part of the left circumflex artery was gently dissected free over a distance of 1.0-1.5 cm proximal of the origin of the first large obtuse marginal branch. A ring-mounted 20 MHz pulsed Doppler probe (Crystal Biotech., Holleston, MA) was placed around the artery and a circular balloon occluder (Jones RE, Silver Spring, MD) was placed just distal to the Doppler probe (figure 6.1). The pericardium and chest were closed and the instrumentation leads were placed in a subcutaneous pocket until the time of study. Long-acting ampicillin 20 mg/kg i.m. was administered one hour prior to the operation and repeated every 48 hours.

Eleven days after instrumentation, each dog was anesthetized by nicomorphine 10 mg/h i.v. and ethrane. No atropine or barbiturates were administered this time. The subcutaneous pocket was opened and the wires of the Doppler probe were connected to the appropriate recording equipment (545C-4 Directional Pulsed Doppler Flow meter, Dept. of Bioengineering, Univ. of Iowa). The pacing electrodes were attached to a trigger unit and the occluder tube was connected to a 5cc syringe. Both femoral arteries were dissected free. An 8F pigtail manometer catheter (Millar microtip catheter transducer SPC-780C) was introduced into the left femoral artery and positioned for simultaneous pressure recording in the left ventricle and the ascending aorta. A 5F left Judkins catheter was introduced into the right femoral artery and advanced into the ostium of the left coronary artery. Once in place, the position of the coronary

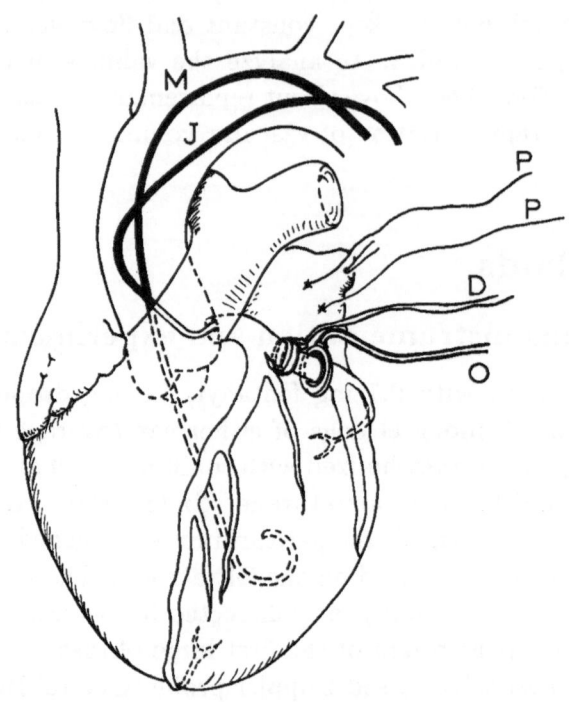

Figure 6.1: *Animal instrumentation. D = Doppler flow velocity probe, J = 5F left Judkins catheter # 3.5, M = Millar pigtail tipmanometer catheter for simultaneous aortic and left ventricular pressure recording, O = Balloon occluder, P = Atrial pacing electrodes.*

catheter was not varied during the study. ECG, left ventricular pressure and its first derivative, aortic pressure, and phasic and mean coronary blood flow velocity in the LCx artery were recorded on an 8-channel recorder (Hewlett Packard). Animal body temperature, carbon dioxide content of end-expiratory air (Gould Goddard Capnograph Mark II) and the fluid balance of the dogs were monitored.

6.2.2 Achievement of constant vascular volume and different flow levels

After intravenous infusion of 5 mg propranolol over 20 minutes to prevent disproportionate increase in heart rate, an initial dose of dipyridamole

of 0.75 mg/kg was administered intravenously during 4 minutes to create maximal dilation of the myocardial vascular bed, followed by 0.1
mg/kg/min for maintenance of this maximal dilated state. Presence of
maximal vasodilation was verified by the absence of any additional flow
increase after 20 seconds of occlusion (figure 6.2) or after intracoronary
administration of 7.5 mg of papaverine. In one dog the dipyridamole
dose had to be doubled before maximal vasodilation occurred. Subsequently the balloon occluder was inflated in 2 series of 6 small steps
guided by the mean Doppler signal and resulting in a step by step decrease of coronary flow velocity (figure 6.2).

6.2.3 Image acquisition and image processing

Image acquisition and processing were performed using a Siemens Bicor
X-ray system connected to a Siemens Digitron-3 computer for digital
subtraction angiography (Siemens AG, Erlangen, FRG). After stabiliza-
tion of the hemodynamic parameters at every degree of stenosis, 6 ml of
contrast agent (iohexol-140, Nycomed) was injected into the left coronary artery, using an angiographic power injector (Sybron Angiomat
300) with an injection rate of 4 ml/s. Flow was not noticeably influenced by the contrast injections (figure 6.2). Contrast injection started
automatically 5 seconds after the start of image acquisition to provide a
stable baseline density level. The moment at which contrast agent ap-
peared in the left main stem was defined as $t = 0$. Voltage and current of
the X-ray generator and pulse width were identical in all studies of one
dog and the automatic brightness control of the equipment was switched
off after the 4th image in every series to enable density comparison within
one study and from one study to another. All studies were performed
using a 7 inch image intensifier. The radiographic projection was chosen
so that the parts of the myocardium corresponding with the left anterior
descending (LAD) and left circumflex (LCx) artery were well separated,
usually the LAO 60° view. Meticulous care was taken not to change
the dog's position during the course of the experiment or allow motion
during image acquisition. Image acquisition was performed in the ECG-
triggered mode using the principle of apparent cardiac arrest [26]. This
means that the heart is stimulated slightly above its inherent frequency
to provide a strictly regular heart rate, that one image is taken per heart
cycle just before onset of the QRS-complex, and that X-rays pulses are
in phase with the cardiac cycle. This is achieved by triggering both the

Figure 6.2: *(next page) Example of step by step stenosis induction in the circumflex artery during maximally dilated - and therefore constant - myocardial vascular volume achieved by continuous dipyridamole infusion.*
ECG, left ventricular pressure (LVP), left ventricular dP/dt (LV dP/dt), aortic pressure (AoP), and phasic and mean Doppler shift are recorded. From left to right, step by step increases in stenosis correspond to step by step decreases in flow velocity. A contrast injection is performed during every flow level and causes an artifactual short dip due to lack of ultrasound reflection by the contrast agent. No increase in flow is observed following contrast injection and flow remains constant during image acquisition. Absence of breathing shortly before and during image acquisition can be recognized in the pressure signals. Presence of maximal vascular volume is confirmed by the absence of any additional hyperemia after 20 seconds of LCx occlusion (right part of the figure). This maximal flow velocity equals the signal obtained in the left part of the figure where no stenosis is present. Note that during steady- state drug infusion no changes in LVP and LV dP/dt are observed. (From Pijls et al., with permission of the American Heart Association, Inc.

pacemaker and the X-ray generator by the videoclock of the image acquisition system. To prevent motion due to breathing the muscle relaxant drug norcuron 0.1 mg/kg/h was administered intravenously, artificial respiration was stopped, and the intratracheal tube was clamped during image acquisition. The last image before contrast injection was taken as a mask and in this way subtraction images without noticeable motion artifacts were acquired during 20-25 consecutive heart cycles. After logarithmic amplification, images were digitized in 512×512 matrices with 1024 density levels using a 10 bit ADC at a rate of 22mHz, and subsequently stored.

6.2.4 Processing of regions of interest and time-density curves

Regions of interest were chosen over the left main stem of the dogs to record the start of contrast injection and over the parts of the myocardium supplied by the LCx artery as well as the LAD artery for myocardial flow assessment (figure 6.3). All ROIs over the myocardium were circular and of identical size (225-400 pixels). Close to the myocardial ROIs (CM_1, CM_2, LM_1 and LM_2), background ROIs (BCM_1,

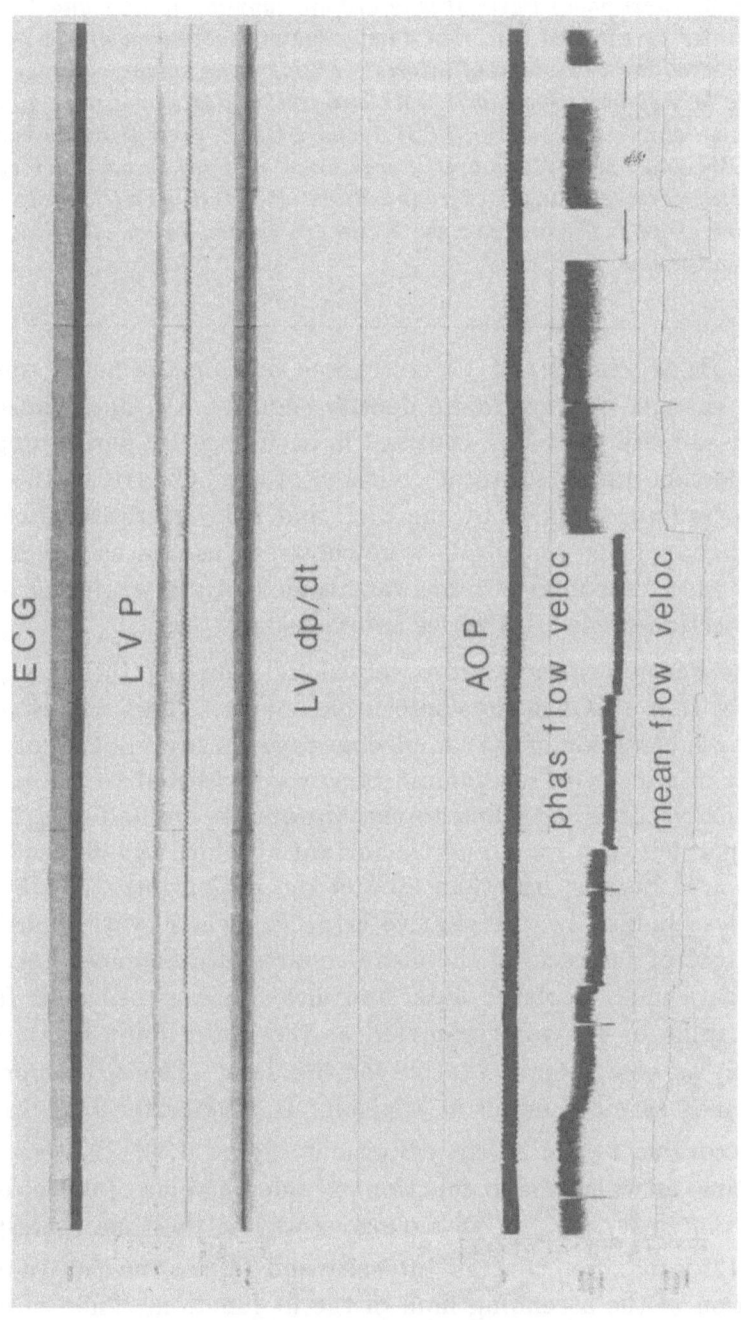

ECG

L V P

LV dp/dt

AOP

phas flow veloc

mean flow veloc

Figure 6.3: *(next page) Parts of myocardium supplied by LCx and LAD artery are separated by contrast injection during subtotal occlusion of the LCx artery (top). Positioning of regions of interest (ROIs) in an image obtained during a moderate LCx stenosis (bottom). CM1 and CM2 : ROIs over myocardium supplied by the circumflex artery. BCM 1 and BCM2: corresponding background ROIs. LM1 and LM2 : ROIs over myocardium supplied by LAD artery. BLM1 and BLM2: corresponding background ROIs. P : ROI over left main stem. In all studies of an individual dog the ROIs are chosen in an identical way and are of similar size.*

BCM_2, BLM_1 and BLM_2) were chosen outside the heart contour to analyze changes in background density (figure 6.3). Once chosen, ROI position and size were kept constant in each dog. By performing a contrast injection during subtotal occlusion of the LCx artery, the parts of the myocardium supplied by the LAD and LCx arteries could be separately distinguished and ROIs were chosen in such a way that overlap of LAD- and LCx-myocardium was avoided. Care was taken to avoid overprojection of visible arteries and veins.

Time density curves were obtained by sampling the average pixel density within a ROI in the consecutive images. These curves were corrected by subtraction of the sampled average densities in the corresponding background ROIs. A gamma function was fitted to the remaining time-density curve according to the Marquardt method [27, 28], using all samples between $t = 0$ and the instant at which the descending part of the curve became less than 60% of the peak value. The quality of the fit was judged by the relative error E_r ,which was defined as the square root of the ratio of the mean squares of differences between observed data and calculated data ,and mean squares of the fit function. A 10% value of E_r was considered as the upper limit for acceptance of the fit as being representative for the data. This fitting procedure is described in more detail in appendix B. Thereafter T_{app} was calculated according to 3 different definitions (figure 6.4): $T_{app}^{(1)}$ was defined as the time at which the fit function exceeded a value of $0.01 \times$ maximal contrast intensity, $T_{app}^{(2)}$ in an analogous way as the time corresponding with $0.125 \times$ maximal contrast intensity and $T_{app}^{(3)}$ as the time of maximal inclination of the ascending limb of the fit function. Time of maximal contrast intensity (T_{max}) was defined as the time corresponding with the top of the fitted curve. T_{mn} was computed directly from the param-

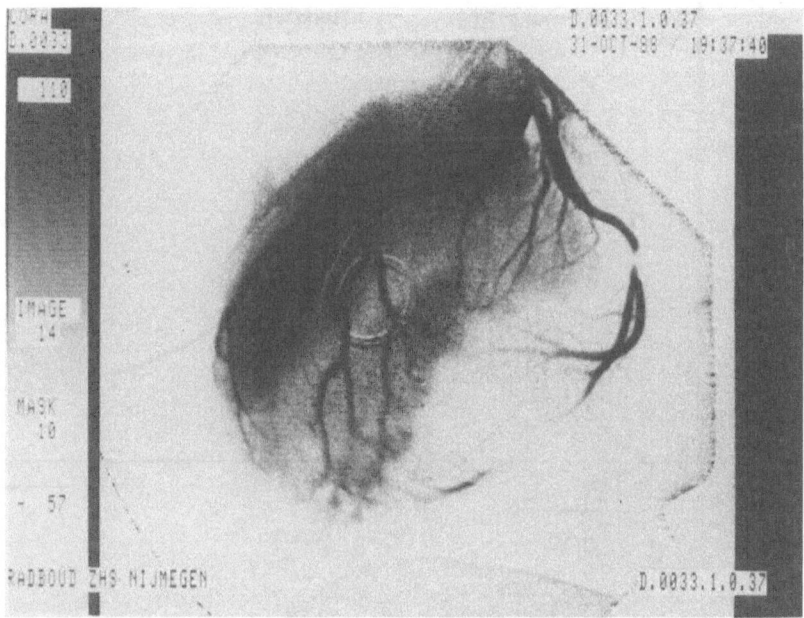

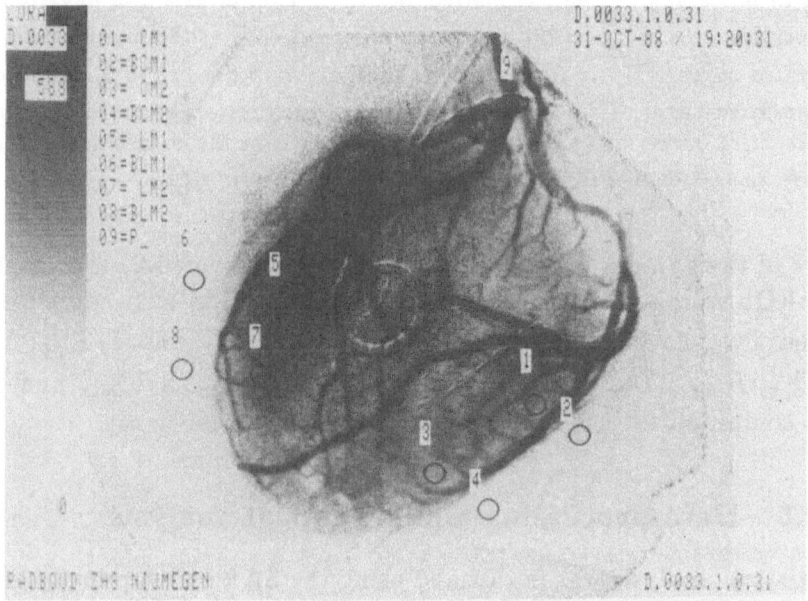

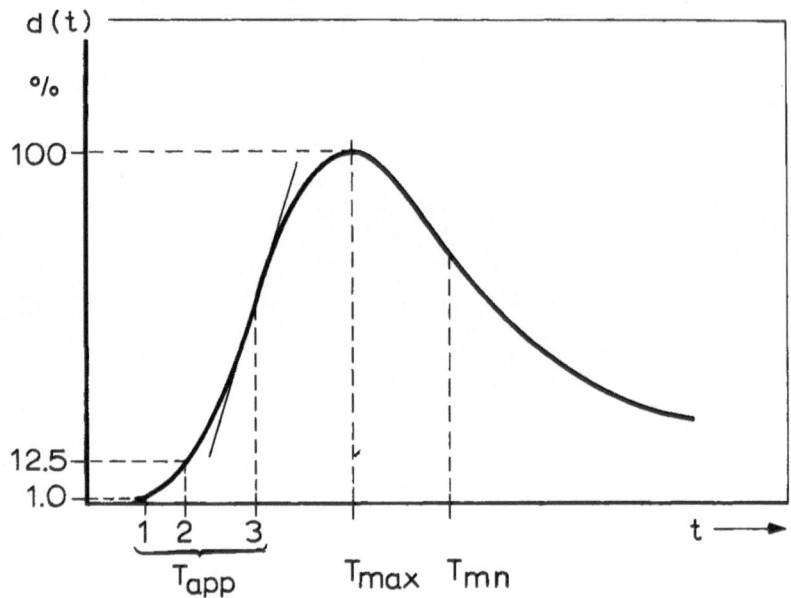

Figure 6.4: *Schematic representation of the definition of time parameters as used in this study. Time t is plotted on the horizontal axis and density d(t) on the vertical axis.* $T_{app}^{(1)}$ = *time corresponding with 1% of the maximal density of the fitted curve,* $T_{app}^{(2)}$ = *time corresponding with 12.5% of the maximal density of the fitted curve,* $T_{app}^{(3)}$ = *time of maximal inclination of the ascending limb of the fitted curve,* T_{max} = *time corresponding with the maximum of the fitted curve,* T_{mn} = *mean transit time as defined in equation (8.2).*

eters of the gamma function according to equation (6.2). For each ROI the ROI-averaged maximal contrast intensity was also computed and called D_{max}. The relation between flow velocity and $1/T_{app}^{(1)}$, $1/T_{app}^{(2)}$, $1/T_{app}^{(3)}$, D_{max}, $D_{max}/T_{app}^{(1)}$, $D_{max}/T_{app}^{(2)}$, $D_{max}/T_{app}^{(3)}$, $1/T_{max}$ and $1/T_{mn}$ was computed for the myocardial ROIs in all dogs.

6.2.5 Data processing and statistical analysis

Statistical analysis was performed using the SAS-software package (SAS Institute Inc, Cary, NC). Hemodynamic data are presented as mean ± standard deviation.

In testing reproducibility of calculation of T_{mn}, in every dog 2 arbitrary studies were performed in duplicate. The correlation coefficients between the first and the second measurement were calculated for the respective ROIs.

According to equation (6.1), the relation between $1/T_{mn}$ and flow and between flow and volume should be linear. Therefore the relations between the inverse time parameters and flow, between D_{max} and flow and between D_{max}/T_{app} and flow were tested on a linear model, according to the F-test. A p-level of < 0.05 was considered to be significant.

The results of the eight dogs will be presented in two ways: 1. For the individual dogs the median and range of correlation coefficients were evaluated for all investigated parameters and for both ROIs belonging to the LCx myocardium. 2. The data of all dogs were normalized and collected in one population. Normalization was performed in every dog by expressing the corresponding time parameter in a particular study as the ratio to the value of this parameter in the study without coronary artery stenosis. Flow velocity was normalized in an analogous way. The linear model was also tested for these normalized data. For the ROIs belonging to the LAD myocardium, only T_{mn} was analyzed. Because the flow in the LAD artery was not directly measured, these values for T_{mn} are corrected for changes in mean arterial pressure.

6.3 Results

6.3.1 Hemodynamic observations and verification of the animal model

The dipyridamole infusion induced maximal flow velocity within 4 minutes in all dogs. Steady-state values for left ventricular pressure, left ventricular dP/dt, aortic pressure and heart rate were reached within 10 minutes in 4 dogs. In the remaining 4 dogs a slight gradual further decrease of arterial pressure occurred during the course of the experiment, accompanied by a similar decrease in coronary flow velocity. In this way a constant (and maximal) vascular volume was achieved during the remaining part of the experiment. This was confirmed by the absence of any increase in flow velocity after 20 seconds of occlusion (figure 6.2) or after intracoronary injections of 7.5 mg papaverine at the start and at the end of a series of studies. Figure 6.2 also shows that contrast injection is not followed by any change in flow velocity and that flow remains constant during image acquisition. The sharp dips are artifacts caused by the rapid passage of the contrast bolus which does not contain particles to reflect ultrasound. After dipyridamole infusion flow velocity increased to $346 \pm 39\%$ of its resting value. This velocity was approximately 15% less than the maximal flow velocity at the start of the experiments, which was due to the decrease of mean arterial pressure during dipyridamole infusion. Maximal Doppler shift was 6.4 ± 0.9 kHz. Calibration against an EM probe was performed succesfully in 6 of the 8 dogs shortly before sacrifice and an excellent correlation between both measurements was found in all cases ($r = 0.96 \pm 0.05$ cf. figure 2.2). Maximal Doppler shift corresponded with a maximal volumetric flow of 174 ± 42 ml/min.

6.3.2   Quality of image acquisition and time-density curves

Almost motionless image acquisition was achieved during 20-25 consecutive heart beats in 91 out of 96 studies (94%). The excellent image quality is demonstrated in figure 6.5 and 6.6. Although the amount of iodine used in this study was 4 times lower than in regular studies, clear visualization of the epicardial coronary arteries, the myocardium itself, and even the coronary venous system was possible.

The positions of the respective myocardial ROIs and their corresponding background ROIs, two over the LCx myocardium and two over the LAD-myocardium, are indicated in figure 6.3. Some examples of time-density curves, the corresponding background curves, the background corrected curves, and the corresponding fits are shown in figure 6.7 and 6.8. After background correction, the baseline is more constant and the descending part of the curve returns to the baseline. Adequate fits could always be obtained. The relative error E_r, representing the quality of the fit, was always less than 10% and on average less than 3%.

Reproducibility of T_{mn} obtained under identical circumstances within one dog was excellent. The correlation coefficients between the first and the second measurement were 0.98, 0.97, 0.91 and 0.96 for the ROI $CM_1, CM_2, LM_1,$ and LM_2 respectively.

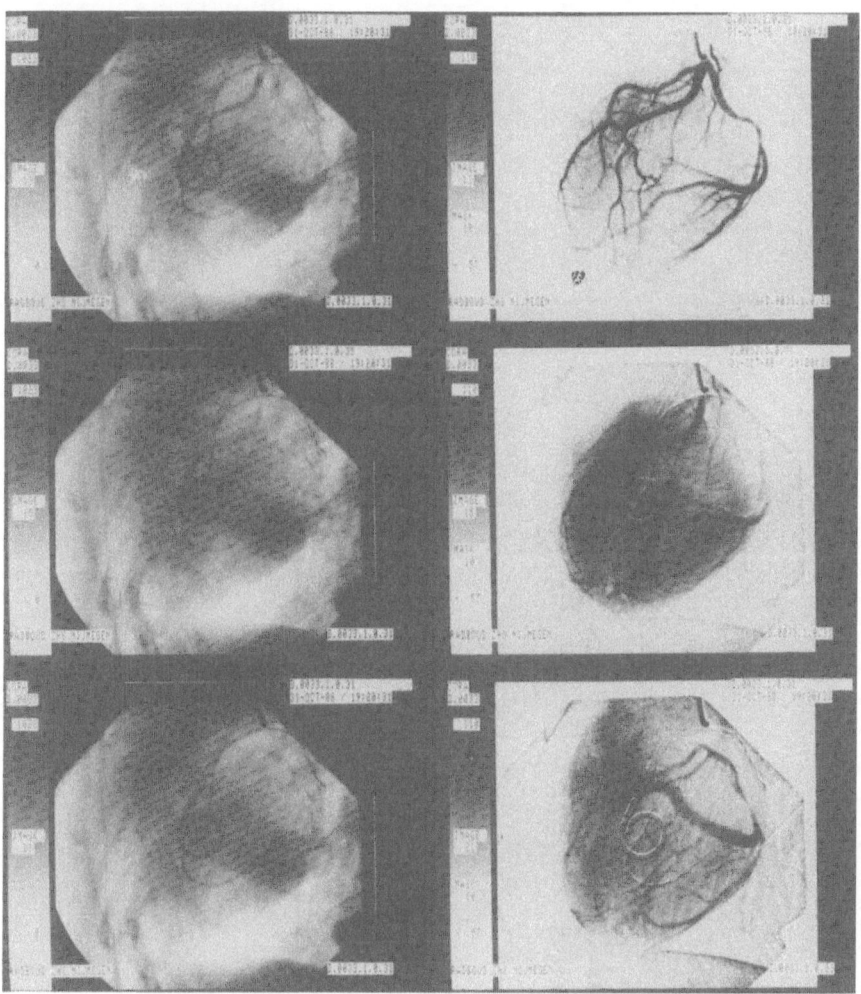

Figure 6.5: *Illustration of the image enhancement achieved in this study. The left series corresponds with the 3rd, 5th and 11th unsubtracted image after contrast injection of 6 ml Iohexol-140. The right series represents the corresponding images using mask mode digital subtraction.*

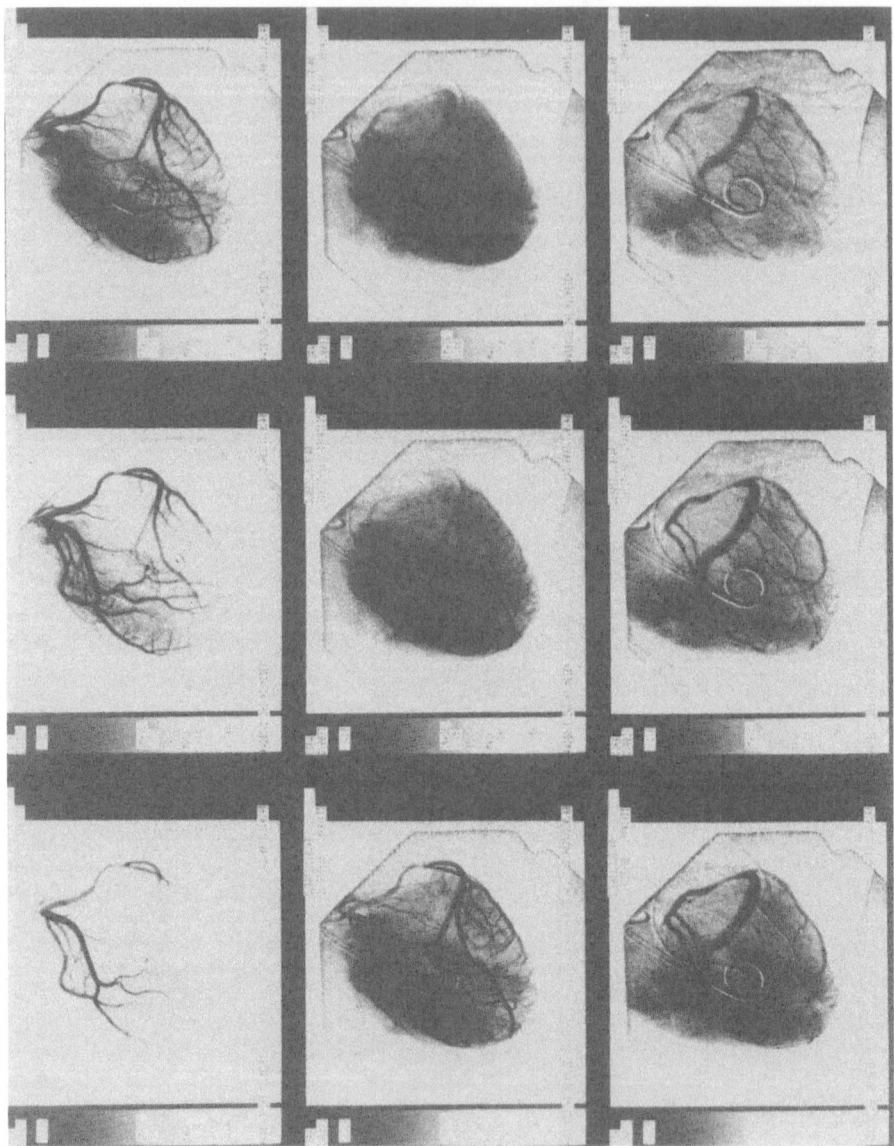

Figure 6.6: *Example of a representative sequence of mask mode subtracted images, obtained during moderate LCx stenosis. Not only the coronary arteries and the myocardial vascular bed are clearly visible, but even the coronary venous system and the right atrium are well delineated. Capillary filling and washout can easily be observed. Even in the last image, 20 heart cycles after the start of image acquisition, motion artifacts are only mild.*

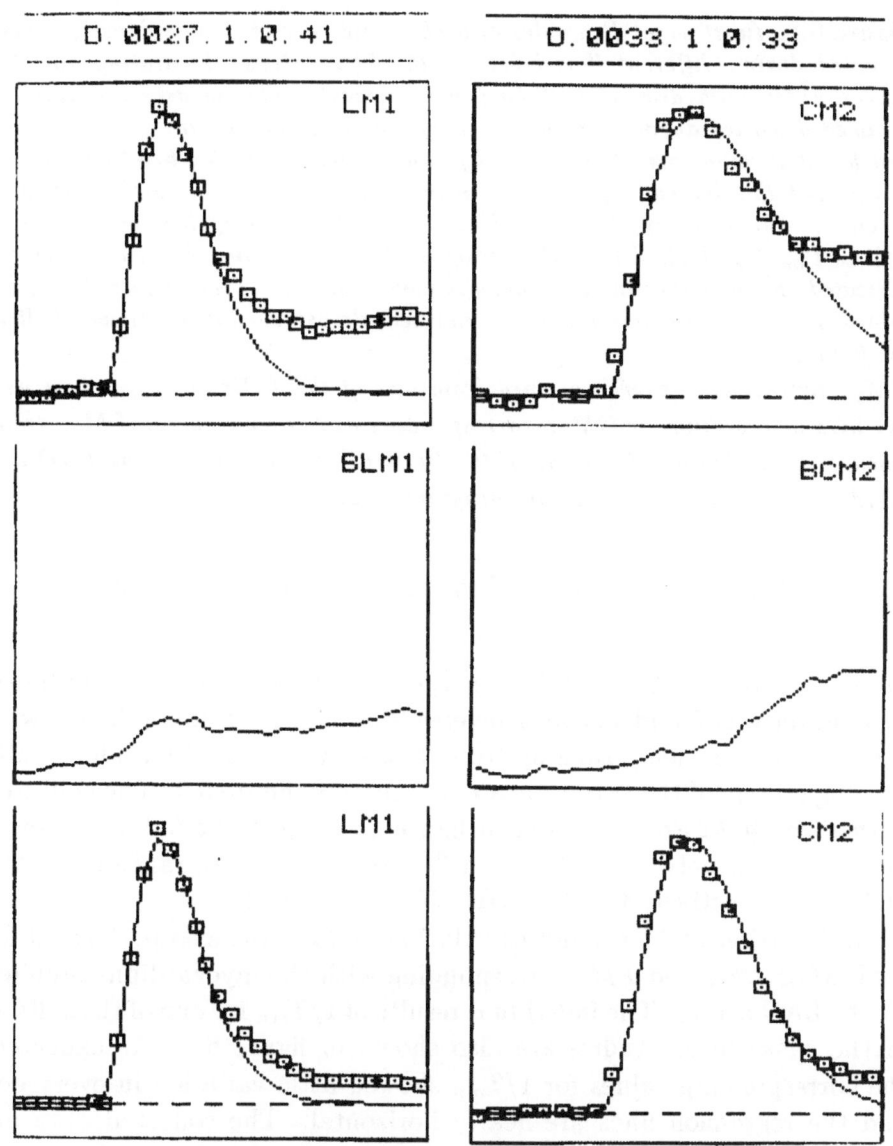

Figure 6.7: *Example of some time-density curves (upper part of the figure), the corresponding background curves (middle part), the background corrected curves (lower part) and the corresponding fits. The sampled densities are indicated by squares and the fits by the dotted lines. Before background correction, the descending part of the TDC shows slow kinetics but after correction for changes in background density this tail returns to the baseline. (From Pijls et al., with permission of the American Heart Association, Inc.)*

Figure 6.8: *(next page) Examples of background corrected time-density curves obtained during different flow levels in the LCx artery, illustrating how the curves widen with decreasing flow (upper series). The squares indicate the sampled densities during subsequent images and the drawn line represents the best fit. Following correction for background density, a stable baseline was obtained and the descending part of the time-density curve almost returned to baseline. The scale on the vertical axis is arbitrary. Doppler shift (kHz) as well as T_{mn} (s), derived from the background corrected time density curves are indicated. Remark that the time-density curves over the LAD myocardium, obtained during the various studies, remained almost unchanged (lower half of the figure).*
CM_2: time-density curve obtained from one of the ROIs corresponding with the LCx myocardium. BCM_2: corresponding background curve. LM_2: time-density curve obtained from one of the ROIs corresponding with the LAD myocardium. BLM_2: corresponding background curve.

6.3.3   Relation between inverse mean transit time and flow

In all dogs and for both ROIs over the LCx myocardium, a good linear correlation was found between inverse T_{mn} and LCx flow velocity with correlation coefficients ranging from 0.92 - 0.99 (table 6.1). The results per dog for one of the two ROIs are presented in figure 6.9. The collected normalized data are presented in figure 6.10 and table 6.2 and show a linear relation between $1/T_{mn}$ and flow over the entire range ($r = 0.94$ and 0.95 respectively for the ROIs CM_1 and CM_2).

Delineation of TDCs and calculation of T_{mn} was also performed for both ROIs LM_1 and LM_2 corresponding with the myocardium supplied by the LAD artery. The individual results of $1/T_{mn}$ for one of these ROIs in the consecutive studies are also shown in figure 6.9. As expected, the corresponding values for $1/T_{mn}$ showed little variation in every dog and the regression lines are nearly horizontal. The collected data are presented in table 6.2.

6.3.4   Relation between $1/T_{app}^{(1)}$, $1/T_{app}^{(2)}$, $1/T_{app}^{(3)}$, D_{max} , $D_{max}/T_{app}^{(1)}$, $D_{max}/T_{app}^{(2)}$, $D_{max}/T_{app}^{(3)}$, $1/T_{max}$ and flow

The relation between $1/T_{app}^{(1)}$, $1/T_{app}^{(2)}$ and $1/T_{app}^{(3)}$ respectively and flow was studied for ROI CM_1 and CM_2 in an analogous way. A linear

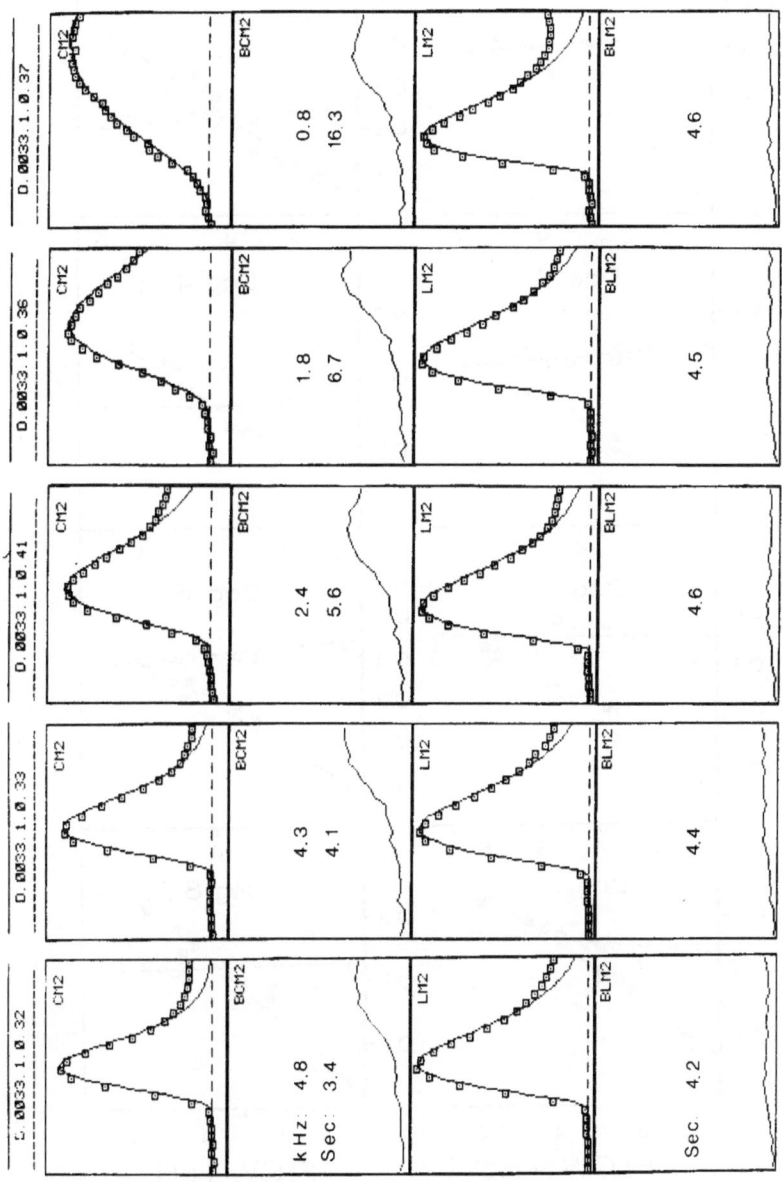

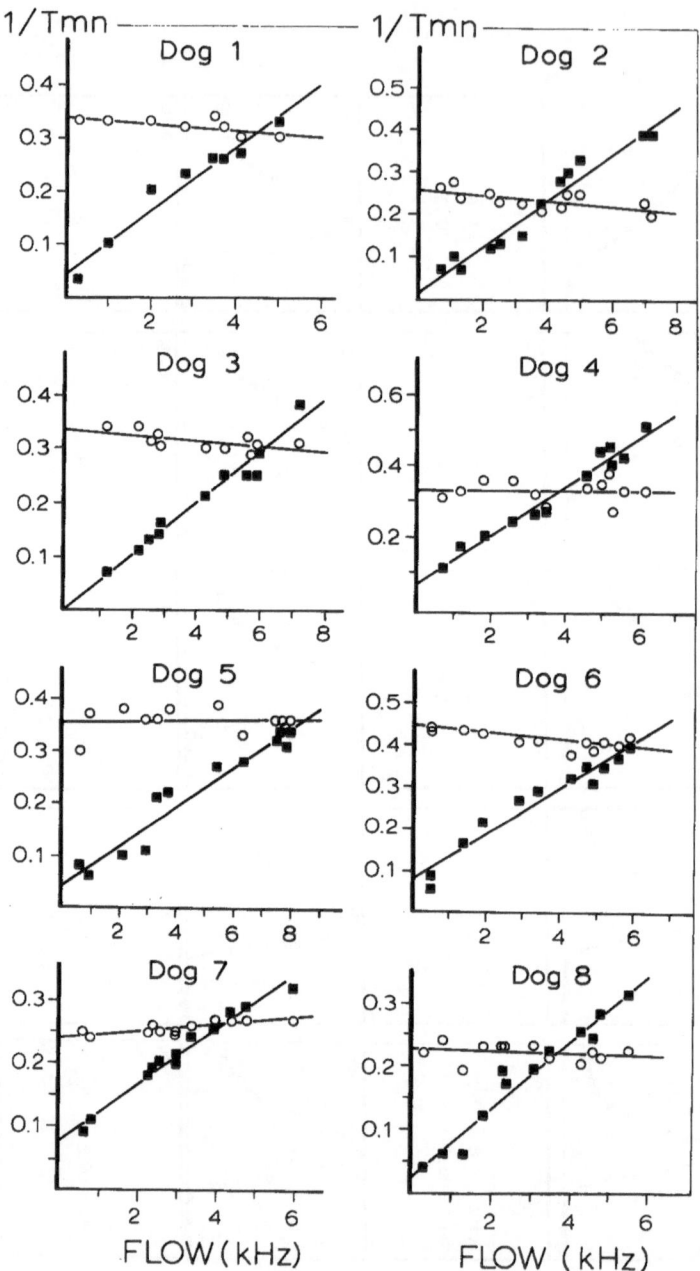

Figure 6.9: *LCx flow velocity vs. inverse mean transit time (1/T_mn) during different degrees of LCx stenosis for the individual dogs for one ROI over the LCx myocardium and one ROI over the LAD myocardium. bold squares = LCx myocardium; open circles = LAD myocardium. (From Pijls et al., with permission of the American Heart Association, Inc.)*

Table 6.1: *Median (r) and range of correlation coefficients for the different investigated parameters for the regions of interest CM_1 and CM_2 over the myocardium supplied by the LCx artery. The number of dogs for which a linear model may be hypothetized according to the F-test, is indicated by m.*

N = 8 dogs	CM_1				CM_2			
	m	r	range		m	r	range	
$1/T_{app}^{(1)}$	2	0.69	0.15 -	0.82	3	0.59	-0.58 -	0.87
$1/T_{app}^{(2)}$	6	0.75	0.26 -	0.91	5	0.67	0.16 -	0.91
$1/T_{app}^{(3)}$	1	0.57	-0.67 -	0.77	4	0.60	-0.60 -	0.93
D_{max}	5	0.80	0.56 -	0.96	5	0.77	0.58 -	0.96
$D_{max}/T_{app}^{(1)}$	5	0.82	0.31 -	0.95	4	0.74	-0.36 -	0.95
$D_{max}/T_{app}^{(2)}$	6	0.88	0.60 -	0.97	7	0.87	0.72 -	0.93
$D_{max}/T_{app}^{(3)}$	5	0.67	-0.26 -	0.99	4	0.65	-0.43 -	0.99
$1/T_{max}$	8	0.94	0.88 -	0.99	8	0.93	0.90 -	0.98
$1/T_{mn}$	8	0.97	0.92 -	0.99	8	0.97	0.95 -	0.99

relation between $1/T_{app}$ and flow could be shown in a minority of dogs and the correlation coefficients cover a wide range (table 6.1).

If D_{max} adequately represented vascular volume, than this parameter would have to remain unchanged during a series of studies. This was not the case. In all dogs D_{max} decreased with decreasing flow (figure 6.11 and table 6.1).

Subsequently the relation between the D_{max}/T_{app} ratio and flow was investigated for $T_{app}^{(1)}$, $T_{app}^{(2)}$ and $T_{app}^{(3)}$. The correlations obtained were better than those obtained using $1/T_{app}$ or D_{max} alone, but considerably less than the results obtained in using mean transit time (figure 6.11 and table 6.1).

Finally the relation between $1/T_{max}$ and flow was examined. A linear relation was present in all dogs (table 6.1). The correlation coefficients are better for T_{mn} than for T_{max} ($p < 0.05$, Wilcoxon test for paired observations). The differences, however, are small and T_{max} is quite favourable as compared to T_{app} (figure 6.11 and table 6.2).

Table 6.2: *Collected data of all dogs, normalized for the investigated parameter and flow.* r = *correlation coefficient.* SE = *standard error of slope and intercept respectively.* SEE = *standard error of estimate.*

Region of interest CM_1					
	N	r	slope ± SE	int ± SE	SEE
$1/T_{app}^{(1)}$	83	0.22	0.97 ± 0.47	0.20 ± 0.30	1.21
$1/T_{app}^{(2)}$	90	0.38	1.18 ± 0.31	0.18 ± 0.20	0.87
$1/T_{app}^{(3)}$	89	0.08	0.29 ± 0.42	0.86 ± 0.29	1.09
D_{max}	91	0.68	0.75 ± 0.09	0.33 ± 0.06	0.25
$D_{max}/T_{app}^{(1)}$	83	0.26	1.47 ± 0.61	-0.15 ± 0.39	0.56
$D_{max}/T_{app}^{(2)}$	90	0.56	1.62 ± 0.25	-0.21 ± 0.16	0.72
$D_{max}/T_{app}^{(3)}$	89	0.47	1.06 ± 0.23	0.15 ± 0.16	0.58
$1/T_{max}$	91	0.93	0.80 ± 0.03	0.26 ± 0.02	0.10
$1/T_{mn}$	91	0.94	0.86 ± 0.03	0.13 ± 0.02	0.09
Region of interest LM_1					
$1/T_{mn}$	86	0.25	0.12 ± 0.05	0.92 ± 0.03	0.14
Region of interest CM_2					
$1/T_{app}^{(1)}$	80	0.22	0.72 ± 0.36	0.12 ± 0.22	0.91
$1/T_{app}^{(2)}$	89	0.41	1.78 ± 0.42	-0.15 ± 0.27	1.20
$1/T_{app}^{(3)}$	90	0.34	1.34 ± 0.43	0.20 ± 0.30	1.03
D_{max}	91	0.72	0.75 ± 0.08	0.30 ± 0.05	0.22
$D_{max}/T_{app}^{(1)}$	80	0.32	0.84 ± 0.28	-0.10 ± 0.17	0.71
$D_{max}/T_{app}^{(2)}$	89	0.45	2.04 ± 0.43	-0.46 ± 0.28	1.23
$D_{max}/T_{app}^{(3)}$	90	0.51	1.62 ± 0.31	-0.20 ± 0.03	0.74
$1/T_{max}$	91	0.90	0.81 ± 0.04	0.26 ± 0.03	0.12
$1/T_{mn}$	91	0.95	0.90 ± 0.03	0.17 ± 0.02	0.09
Region of interest LM_2					
$1/T_{mn}$	90	0.26	0.09 ± 0.03	0.85 ± 0.02	0.10

6.4   Discussion

The experimental model used in this study was devised to be as close to ideal for application of the indicator dilution theory as possible in a living being, using regular catheterization techniques and equipment.

Flow was not influenced by contrast injection and remained constant during the acquisition of the TDC while vascular volume, although unknown, remained unchanged between the different studies (figure 6.2). The presence of a constant and maximal vascular volume was confirmed by lack of additional hyperemia after a 20 second occlusion and after intracoronary papaverine injections.

Image quality was enhanced considerably and passage of contrast through the myocardium supplied by the LCx artery or the LAD artery was studied reliably during 20-25 consecutive heart beats. This resulted in TDCs representing the sampled density values during consecutive heart beats on a scale of 0-1023 density units. This scale is relative and variable from one animal to another. Within one dog, however, this scale is uniform. For all regions of interest, changes in density in corresponding background ROIs outside the left ventricular contour were also analyzed (figure 6.3). This background density usually showed slight variations over time, predominantly an increase. These variations in brightness are caused by the intrinsic instability of the X-ray chain, motion artifacts, and overlap of extramyocardial vascular structures which are stained by contrast during the later phase of image acquisition. By correcting for these changes in background density, the time-density curves almost invariably returned to the baseline. This may explain why in many former studies the TDC failed to return to the baseline, thereby precluding accurate measurement of mean transit time [18, 19, 29].

Because time-density curves in this study were constructed by sampling the average pixel density within the ROI and not on a pixel by pixel basis, this approach does not permit generation of parametric images, but is less influenced by image noise.

After adequate fitting of the background corrected TDC [27, 28], and in the presence of constant vascular volume, reliable and reproducible determination of mean transit time was possible. In all dogs and for both ROIs over the LCx myocardium an excellent correlation was demonstrated between $1/T_{mn}$ and flow (figure 6.9 and 6.10). Moreover, TDCs and T_{mn} belonging to the ROIs over the LAD myocardium, showed only minor changes during progressive flow reduction in the LCx artery,

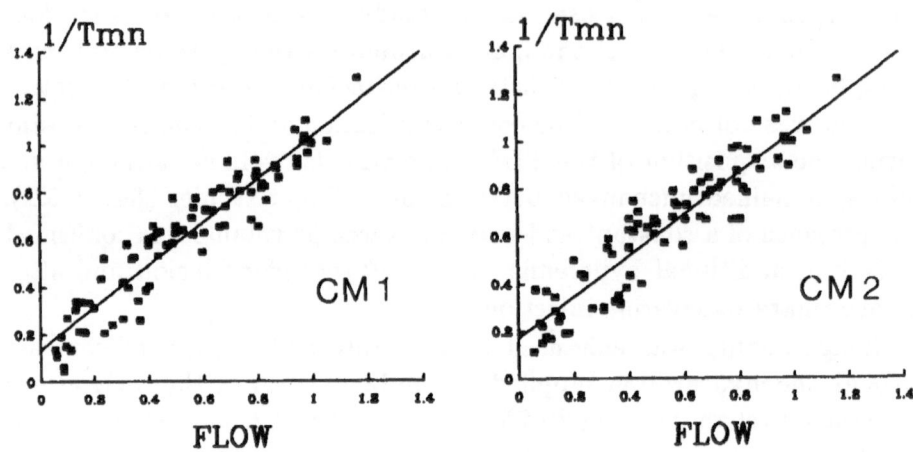

Figure 6.10: *Normalized LCx flow velocity vs. normalized 1/T_{mn} for two ROIs corresponding with the myocardium supplied by the LCx artery.*

which argues for the intrinsic correctness of this model (figure 6.9).

The moment of the first appearance of contrast agent in a region of interest over the proximal part of the left coronary artery, was chosen as t=0. Theoretically, it would have been better to define the mean transit time of the block shaped input signal as t=0, i.e. the moment 0.75 s after start of contrast injection, as has been done in the later human studies (cf. figure 8.1). Because, however, in this animal study also appearance time in the myocardial ROIs was investigated, negative values for this parameter would have been found in that case. If the moment 0.75 s after start of contrast injection would have been taken as t=0, the relation between mean transit time and flow would have been even better in comparison with the present definition.

In this study the gold standard for estimation of flow was the Doppler shift as measured by the epicardial ring mounted Doppler probe. It has been shown numerous times, including in this study, that in the absence of changes in vessel diameter a reliable measure for flow is provided by this method [30, 31, 32, 33].

Our model also offered an ideal opportunity to study the value of other time parameters proposed for myocardial flow assessment and of D_{max} for volume estimation. For the three different definitions of con-

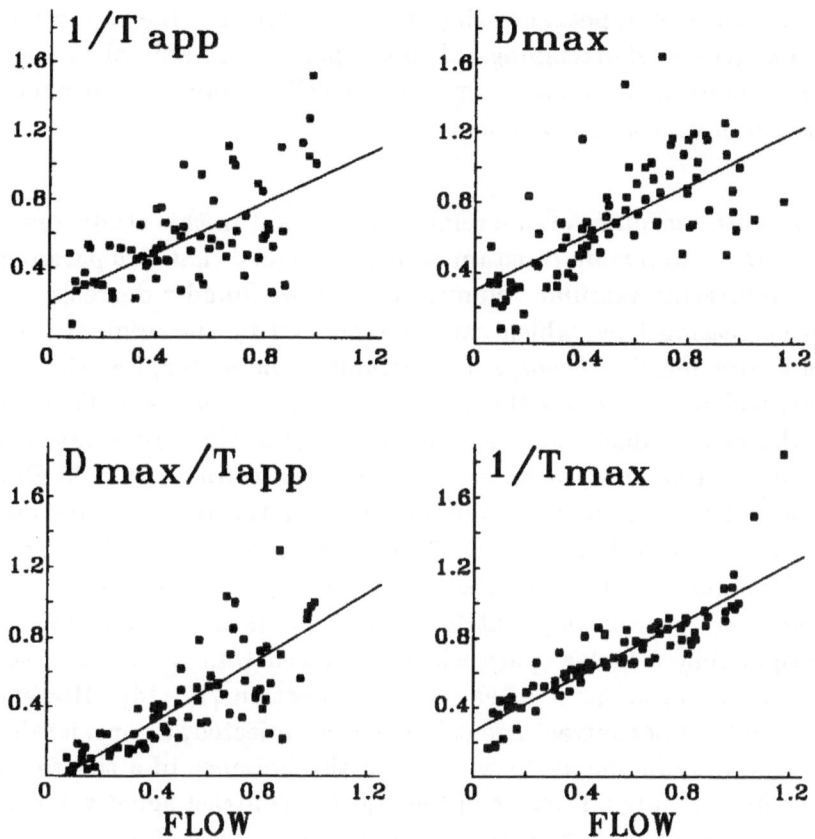

Figure 6.11: *Normalized LCx flow velocity vs. $1/T_{app}^{(2)}$, $D_{max}/T_{app}^{(2)}$, D_{max} and $1/T_{max}$ for one of the ROIs corresponding with the LCx myocardium (CM1). For abbreviations see figure 6.4. Of all 3 definitions used for appearance time, $T_{app}^{(2)}$ was the most favourable.*

trast appearance time used in this study, the relation with flow velocity is rather weak. Although appearance time is differently defined by different authors [9, 10, 12, 13, 15, 16], this time parameter always refers to a moment early in the ascending limb of the TDC. Therefore it is not very likely that the results for inverse appearance time in relation to flow would have been much better in these cases than when using the definitions of appearance time as in the present study.

A poor correlation between appearance time and flow has been documented in some previous studies [13, 17, 34]. It is unlikely that the poorer results of appearance time to assess flow are due to methodological mistakes or shortcomings of this experimental animal model, since the results for mean transit time were excellent and in accordance with standard indicator dilution theory.

Because vascular volume remained constant in this study, one would expect D_{max} to remain constant as well, provided that this parameter reliably represents vascular volume. Instead, we found a decrease of D_{max} with decreasing flow, which can be explained by the original principles of indicator dilution theory. The volume of indicator, i.e. the contrast agent, will pass through the vascular compartment as a dispersed bolus, the rate of dispersion increasing with the time after injection [6]. Because at low flow the moment of passage through a fixed ROI will be later than at high flow, this means that the time density curve at these low flows will be broader and have a lower peak [6]. Justification for replacement of vascular volume by D_{max} in equation 1 has been defended by postulating that for every pixel in a ROI all blood in the corresponding vascular space will be replaced totally by contrast agent at least at one moment after contrast injection [12, 14]. However, although 6-8 ml of contrast agent is generally injected, a considerable part will leak away in the aorta whereas in the presence of a severe stenosis in one branch only a fraction of the injected contrast agent will enter the diseased branch and stain the corresponding myocardium. In addition, according to pathologic studies the maximal volume of the vascular compartment of the heart is approximately 20 ml/100 g [35, 36, 37, 38] and while the vascular volume per unit increases from the left main coronary artery down to the capillary bed, the contrast bolus is actually dispersing. Therefore it appears unlikely that undiluted contrast agent will pass through a myocardial ROI at sites more distal to the injection site. Whatever the explanation may be, D_{max} does not adequately represent vascular volume.

The ratio D_{max}/T_{app} generally showed a better correlation with flow than either components alone for all 3 definitions of T_{app} (figure 6.11 and table 6.1). It must be emphasized from our results that this improvement is not due to the suitability of D_{max} as an index of vascular volume, but rather that D_{max} is an independent parameter that reflects flow. Accordingly, D_{max}/T_{app} shows a better correlation with flow.

6.5 Clinical implications and limitations

For clinical use this model has some limitations. The patient must stop breathing and remain motionless during at least 15 seconds which requires extensive training. If T_{mn} cannot be determined reliably, use of T_{max}, only slightly less suitable than T_{mn} in this study, could be considered.

Our model is valid in situations of maximal vasodilation to guarantee constant vascular volume. Therefore, it should be emphasized that no information about resting flow can be obtained and that coronary flow reserve cannot be calculated. However, our approach does offer the ability to compare maximal myocardial blood flow before and after an appropriate intervention such as angioplasty or bypass surgery [39]. Unlike coronary flow reserve, this maximal flow ratio is independent of resting flow which in turn is influenced by heart rate, arterial pressure, left ventricular hypertrophy, previous infarction, prolonged ischemia, or by the preceding PTCA procedure itself [25, 39, 40, 41, 42, 43, 44].

Thus, despite potential clinical limitations, this study contributes to the understanding of the methods used to assess myocardial perfusion by studying contrast passage and shows that accurate calculation of relative myocardial perfusion by videodensitometry can be performed in the intact organism according to the original principles of indicator dilution theory.

References

[1] Rutishauser W, Simon H, Stucky J P, Schad N, Noseda G, and Wellauer J. Evaluation of roentgen cinedensitometry for flow measurement in models and in the intact circulation. *Circulation*, 36:951–963, 1967.

[2] Rutishauser W, Bussmann W D, Noseda G, Meier W, and Wellauer J. Blood flow measurement through single coronary arteries by roentgen densitometry. part I: A comparison of flow measured by a radiologic technique applicable in the intact organism and by electromagnetic flowmeter. *Am J Roentgenol*, 109:12–20, 1970.

[3] Rutishauser W, Noseda G, Bussman W D, and Preter B. Blood flow measurement through single coronary arteries by roentgen densitometry. Part II: Right coronary artery flow in conscious man. *Am J Roentgenol*, 109:21–24, 1970.

[4] Smith H C, Sturm R E, and Wood E H. Videodensitometric system for measurement fo vessel blood flow, particularly in the coronary arteries, in man. *Am J Cardiol*, 32:144–150, 1973.

[5] Robb R A, Wood E H, Ritman E L, Johnson S A, Sturm R E, Greenleaf J F, Gilbert B K, and Chevalier P A. Three-dimensional reconstruction and display of the working canine heart and lungs by multiplanar x-ray scanning videodensitometry. In *Computers in Cardiology 1974*, pages 151–163. IEEE Computer Society, Long Beach, 1974.

[6] Zierler K L. *Circulation times and the theory of indicator dilution methods for determining blood flow and volume*, pages 585–615. American Physiological Society, Washington DC, 1962.

[7] Gould K L, Lipscomb K, and Hamilton G W. Physiologic basis for assessing critical coronary stenosis: instantaneous flow response and regional distribution during coronary hyperemia as measures of coronary flow reserve. *Am J Cardiol*, 33:87–94, 1974.

[8] Gould K L and Lipscomb K. Effects of coronary stenosis on coronary flow reserve and resistance. *Am J Cardiol*, 34:48–55, 1974.

[9] Vogel R, LeFree M, Bates E, O'Neill W, Foster R, Kirlin P, Smith D, and Pitt B. Application of digital techniques to selective coronary arteriography: use of myocardial appearance time to measure coronary flow reserve. *Am Heart J*, 107:153–164, 1984.

[10] Vogel R A, Bates E R, O'Neill W W, Aueron F M, Meier B, and Gruentzig A R. Coronary flow reserve measured during cardiac catheterization. *Arch Intern Med*, 144:1773–1776, 1984.

[11] Hodgson J M, Legrand V, Bates E R, Mancini G B J, Aueron F M, O'Neill W W, Simon S B, Beauman G J, LeFree M T, and Vogel R A. Validation in dogs of a rapid digital angiographic technique to measure relative coronary blood flow during routine cardiac catheterization. *Am J Cardiol*, 55:188–193, 1985.

[12] Vogel R A. Radiographic assessment of coronary blood flow parameters. *Circulation*, 72:460–465, 1985.

[13] Bates E R, Aueron F M, Legrand V, LeFree M T, Mancini G B J, Hodgson J M, and Vogel R A. Comparative long-term effects of coronary artery bypass graft surgery and percutaneous transluminal coronary angioplasty on regional coronary flow reserve. *Circulation*, 72:833–839, 1985.

[14] Cusma J T, Toggart E J, Folts J D, Peppler W W, Hagiandreou N J, Lee C S, and Mistretta C A. Digital subtraction imaging of coronary flow reserve. *Circulation*, 75:461–472, 1987.

[15] Zijlstra F, Den Boer A, Reiber J H C, Van Es G A, Lubsen J, and Serruys P W. Assessment of immediate and long-term results of percutaneous transluminal coronary angioplasty. *Circulation*, 78:15–24, 1988.

[16] Spiller P, Schmiel F K, Politz B, Block M, Fermor U, Hackbarth W, Jehle J, Korfer R, and Pannek H. Measurement of systolic and diastolic flow rates in the coronary artery system by x-ray videodensitometry. *Circulation*, 68:337–347, 1983.

[17] Ikeda H, Koga Y, Utsu F, and Toshima H. Quantitative evaluation of regional myocardial blood flow by videodensitometric analysis of digital subtraction coronary arteriography in humans. *J Am Coll Cardiol*, 8:809–816, 1986.

[18] Nishimura R A, Rogers P J, Holmes D R, Gehring D G, and Bove A A. Assessment of myocardial perfusion by videodensitometry in the canine model. *J Am Coll Cardiol*, 9:891–897, 1987.

[19] Toggart E J and Mistretta C A. Digital coronary angiography: approaches using intravenous and direct methods. In G B J Mancini, editor, *Clinical applications of cardiac digital angiography*, pages 253–279. Raven Press, New York, 1988.

[20] Van der Werf T, Heethaar R M, Stegehuis H, Pijls N H J, and Meijler F L. *Comparison of time parameters derived from myocardial time-density curves in patients before and after percutaneous transluminal coronary angioplasty*, pages 227–236. Martinus Nijhoff, Dordrecht, Lancaster, Boston, 1988.

[21] Whiting J S, Drury J K, Pfaff J M, Chang B L, Eigler N L, Meerbaum S, Corday E, Nivatpumin T, Forrester J S, and Swan H J C. Digital angiographic measurement of radiographic contrast material kinetics for estimation of myocardial perfusion. *Circulation*, 73:789–798, 1986.

[22] Legrand V, Hodgson J M, Bates E R, Aueron F M, Mancini G B J, Smith J S, Gross M D, and Vogel R A. Abnormal coronary flow reserve and abnormal radionuclide excercise test results in patient with normal coronary angiograms. *J Am Coll Cardiol*, 6:1245–1253, 1985.

[23] Zijlstra F, Reiber J C, Juilliere Y, and Serruys P W. Normalizaiton of coronary flow reserve by percutaneous transluminal coronary angioplasty. *Am J Cardiol*, 61:55–60, 1988.

[24] Serruys P W, Zijlstra F, Juilliere Y, De Feyter P J, Van den Brand M, Suryapranata H, and Reiber J H C. *How to assess the immediate results of PTCA. Should we use pressure gradient, flow reserve or minimal luminal cross-sectional area?*, pages 181–206. Kluwer Academic Publishers, Dordrecht, 1988.

[25] O'Neill W W, Walton J A, Bates E R, Colfer H T, Aueron F M, LeFree M T, Pitt B, and Vogel R A. Criteria for successful coronary angioplasty as assessed by alterations in coronary vasodilatory reserve. *J Am Coll Cardiol*, 3:1382–1390, 1984.

[26] Van der Werf T, Heethaar R M, Stegehuis H, and Meijler F L. The concept of apparent cardiac arrest as a prerequisite for coronary digital subtraction angiography. *J Am Coll Cardiol*, 4:239–244, 1984.

[27] Bevington P R. *Data reduction and error analysis for the physical sciences*, pages 204–246. McGraw-Hill, New York, 1969.

[28] Uijen G H J, Pijls N H J, and Van der Werf T. The accuracy of densitometric time parameters in the analysis of myocardial perfusion. In *Computers in Cardiology 1988*, pages 215–218. IEEE Computer Society, Washington DC, 1989.

[29] Nissen S E, Elion J L, Booth D C, Evans J, and DeMaria A N. Value and limitations of computer analysis of digital subtraction angiography in the assessment of coronary flow reserve. *Circulation*, 73:562–571, 1986.

[30] Marcus M, Wright C, Doty D, Eastham C, Laughlin D, Krumm P, Fastenow C, and Brody M. Measurements of coronary velocity and reactive hyperemia in the coronary circulation of humans. *Circ Res*, 49:877–891, 1981.

[31] Vatner S F, Franklin D, and Vancitters R L. Simultaneous comparison and calibration of the Doppler and electromagnetic flowmeters. *J Appl Physiol*, 29:907–910, 1970.

[32] Hartley C J and Cole J S. An ultrasonic pulsed Doppler system for measuring blood flow in small vessels. *J Appl Physiol*, 37:626–629, 1974.

[33] Haywood J R, Shaffer R A, Fastenow C, Fink G D, and Brody M J. Regional blood flow measurement with pulsed Doppler flowmeter in conscious rat. *Am J Physiol*, 241:H273–H278, 1981.

[34] Pijls N H J. Meting van de doorbloeding van het myocard. *Cardioselecta*, 7:1–16, 1989.

[35] Crystal G J, Downey H F, and Bashour F A. Small vessel and total coronary blood volume during intracoronary adenosine. *Am J Physiol*, 241:H194–H201, 1981.

[36] Weiss H R and Winbury M M. Nitroglycerine and chromonar on small-vessel content of the ventricular walls. *Am J Physiol*, 226:838–843, 1974.

[37] O'Keefe D D, Hoffman J I E, Cheitlin R, O'Neill M J, Allard J R, and Shapkin E. Coronary blood flow in experimental canine left ventricular hyperthrophy. *Circ Res*, 43:43–51, 1978.

[38] Bassingthwaighte J B, Yipinstoi T, and Harvey R B. Microvasculature of the dog left ventricular myocardium. *Microvasc Res*, 7:229–249, 1974.

[39] Gould K L. Identifying and measuring severity of coronary artery stenosis. Quantitative coronary arteriography and positron emission tomography. *Circulation*, 78:237–245, 1988.

[40] Hoffman J I E. Maximal coronary flow and the concept of coronary vascular reserve. *Circulation*, 70:153–159, 1984.

[41] White C W, Wright C B, Doty D B, Hiratza L F, Eastham C L, Harrison D G, and Marcus M L. Does visual interpretation of the coronary arteriogram predict the physiological importance of a coronary stenosis? *N Engl J Med*, 310:819–824, 1984.

[42] Klein L W, Agarwal J B, Schneider R M, Hermann G, Weintraub W S, and Helfant R H. Effects of previous myocardial infarction on measurements of reactive hyperemia and the coronary vascular reserve. *J Am Coll Cardiol*, 8:357–363, 1986.

[43] Klocke F J. Measurements of coronary flow reserve: defining pathophysiology versus making decisions about patient care. *Circulation*, 76:1183–1189, 1987.

[44] Serruys P W, Juilliere Y, Zijlstra F, Beatt K J, De Feyter P J, Suryapranata H, Van den Brand M, and Roelandt J. Coronary blood flow velocity during percutaneous transluminal coronary angioplasty as a guide for assessment of the functional result. *Am J Cardiol*, 61:253–259, 1988.

Chapter 7

The Concept of Maximal Flow Ratio for Immediate Evaluation of PTCA Result

7.1 Introduction

For many years it has been widely recognized that the best way to evaluate the functional result of a coronary angioplasty is to investigate its effect on coronary flow or myocardial perfusion [1, 2, 3]. One method for flow measurement used in clinical practice nowadays is ECG-triggered digital radiography. Most approaches in this field, however, have at least 3 important limitations, namely 1. the influence of the indicator (contrast agent) on flow, 2. the changes in vascular volume between different situations in which flow is compared, and 3. the limited time available for motionless image acquisition. To avoid these problems, different adjusted versions of the original theory have been proposed with somewhat disappointing results [4, 5, 6, 7, 8, 9, 10, 11]. In fact, most problems are related to the inability to determine resting flow accurately, which implies unreliable assessment of coronary flow reserve [9, 12, 13, 14].

In chapter 6 we described a videodensitometric method for comparison of merely maximal myocardial perfusion between different situations, e.g. different degrees of coronary artery stenosis [15].

In this approach the influence of indicator on flow and changes in vascular volume are circumvented and although no data about resting flow or CFR can be obtained, maximal flow could be determined very accurately in animal validation studies. This method uses mean transit time (T_{mn}) as a single parameter which is inversely proportional to max-

101

imal flow and is strictly in accordance with the mathematical principles
of indicator dilution theory. Considering the fact that in the majority of patients, anginal complaints are not caused by inadequate resting
flow but by impaired maximal flow, it seems to be plausible that the
increase in maximal flow after an intervention will be a straightforward
parameter to reflect functional improvement of the patient [14, 16].

Aims of this study were to test the applicability of this method in
man during PTCA, to relate the relative increase in maximal flow immediately after PTCA to functional improvement at noninvasive exercise
testing 7-10 days later, and to investigate values for mean transit time
during maximal hyperemia in normal coronary arteries.

7.2   Methods

7.2.1   Patient population and study design

Forty consecutive patients, referred for elective PTCA, were included
into this study, who met the following criteria: 1. The presence of the
combination of angina pectoris NYHA class III, a positive exercise test
(ET) and single vessel disease at coronary arteriography at the time of
acceptance for PTCA less than 6 weeks before the actual date of the
intervention; 2. presence of sinus rhythm; 3. absence of previous bypass
surgery or myocardial infarction causing more than mild hypokinesia of
one of the segments on the left ventriculogram; 4. absence of visible
collateral circulation.

These patients were seen at the outpatients' department 24-48 hours
before the intervention. At that time the aim of the study was explained to the patient and another ET was performed. In case of pre-
existent ECG-abnormalities interfering with regular evaluation of the
stress ECG, the test was combined with thallium scintigraphy. This
was the case in only two patients. This ET was followed by extensive
training to hold breath at maximal inspiration for 15-20 seconds, using
a nose clamp. Patients were asked to repeat this training at night and
the next day, lying in the same position as during the catheterization.
Careful attention was paid to avoid motion of head, neck, shoulders and
thorax during the holding of breath.

Exercise testing was repeated 7-10 days after the PTCA. All ETs
were performed on a bicycle ergometer in upright position according to
local routine, starting at a load of 50 W and with a stepwise increase of

10 W/min. A 12-lead ECG was recorded every minute. ET results were classified as negative or mildly, moderately or strongly positive according to Selzer et al.[17]. Thallium scintigraphy was classified as positive, if evident filling defects were present by visual interpretation in at least 2 segments immediately after exercise and had disappeared 4 hours later [18]. All patients used aspirin 160 mg daily and dipyridamole 75 mg q.i.d. from at least 2 days before until 10 days after the procedure. No further restrictions were made concerning concomitant medication.

At the time of the PTCA, a 6 F stimulation catheter was positioned in the right atrium, whereafter the following protocol was performed: In case of a stenosis in one of the large branches of the left coronary artery (LCA), a 7 F diagnostic right Judkins catheter was advanced into the right coronary artery (RCA) and an ECG-triggered digital study was performed in the 30° right anterior oblique projection during maximal vasodilation of the myocardial vascular bed. After changing the coronary catheter, this was followed by a similar study of the LCA in the 60° left anterior oblique projection, sometimes with slight cranial angulation depending on the patient's anatomy. After removal of the diagnostic catheter, an appropriate 8 F guiding catheter was advanced into the LCA. Thereafter the regular PTCA procedure was performed, using preferably an over-the-wire balloon (USCI Simplus, C.R. Bard Ireland Ltd, Galway, Ireland) to enable measurement of transstenotic pressure gradients prior to the first and 5 minutes after the final balloon inflation and at least 2 minutes after intracoronary injection of contrast medium. Fifteen minutes after the last balloon inflation, another ECG- triggered digital study of the LCA during maximal vasodilation was performed using the left Judkins diagnostic catheter. In case of a right coronary artery stenosis, RCA and LCA were interchanged in this protocol. During image acquisition, arterial pressure was recorded continuously through the side channel of the arterial sheath. The stimulated heart rate remained constant in all studies within one patient. By following this protocol, not only data about maximal flow in the diseased artery before and after PTCA could be compared, but in addition reference data for apparently normal coronary arteries could be collected.

7.2.2 Image acquisition and processing

Image acquisition and processing were performed using a Siemens Bicor X-ray system connected to a Siemens Digitron-3 computer for digital subtraction angiography (Siemens AG, Erlangen, FRG). For all studies 6 ml of the nonionic contrast agent Iohexol-350 (Nycomed AS, Oslo, Norway) was injected, using a power injector at a speed of 4 ml/s. Image acquisition was performed during the holding of breath at maximal inspiration as described above and using the principle of apparent cardiac arrest. This means that not only the heart itself is triggered slightly above its inherent frequency to provide a strictly regular heart rhythm, but also that the X-ray pulses are in synchrony with the paced heart beats [19]. One image was obtained per heart cycle, just before the onset of the QRS-complex. Image acquisition started exactly 25 seconds after intracoronary administration of 8 mg of papaverine in the RCA or 12 mg in the LCA to provide maximal vasodilation of the myocardial vascular bed. Contrast injection started 5 sec after the onset of image acquisition to provide a stable baseline density level. The moment at which 50% of the contrast agent was injected, was defined as $t = 0$ (cf figure 8.1). Voltage and current of the X-ray generator and pulse width were identical in all studies within one patient and the automatic brightness control of the X-ray equipment was switched off after the 4th image in every study to enable density comparison within one study. All studies were performed using a 7 inch image intensifier. Meticulous care was taken to avoid changes in the patient's position between the different studies. After logarithmic transformation, images were digitized in a 512×512 matrix with 1024 density levels using a 10 bits ADC at a rate of 22 MHz, and subsequently stored. Stenosis severity before and after the PTCA was assessed by quantitative coronary arteriography, by calculation of the reduction of cross-sectional area as compared to a nearby normal arterial segment (Digitron Stenosis program [20], Siemens AG, Erlangen, FRG).

7.2.3   Processing of the regions of interest and time-density curves.

Regions of interest (ROIs) were chosen over the tip of the coronary catheter to record start of contrast injection and over the myocardium supplied by the respective arteries. For the left anterior descending (LAD) artery, the myocardial ROI was preferably chosen over the antero-apical region, for the left circumflex (LCx) artery over the posterolateral area at the level of the posteromedian papillary muscle and for the RCA over the central portion of the posterior septum (figure 7.1). All myocardial ROIs were circular and of identical size (225-600 pixels) within one patient. ROIs were chosen in such a way that overlap of LAD and LCx myocardium was avoided and care was taken to avoid overprojection of the large epicardial arteries and veins. Close to the myocardial ROIs, background ROIs were chosen for analysis of changes in background density. This analysis is performed because the background always shows slight variations in density over time, predominantly a slight increase. This is caused by instability of the X-ray chain, small motion artifacts, and sometimes overlap of extramyocardial structures such as the descending aorta or the right atrium, which are faintly stained by contrast agent during the latter phase of image acquisition [15]. Once chosen, position and size of the ROIs were kept constant within each patient.

Time density curves were obtained by sampling the average pixel density within a ROI in the consecutive images and corrected by subtraction of the sampled average density in the corresponding background ROI. A gamma function was fitted to the remaining data according to the Marquardt method [21, 22, 23], using all samples between $t = 0$ and the instant at which the descending part of the curve became less than 60% of the peak value.

A 10% value of the relative error E_r was considered as the upper limit for acceptance of the fit as being representative for the sampled data. This is in analogy with the former animal validation study [15, 24, 25]. Mean transit time (T_{mn}) was calculated from the fit function $d(t)$ according to theory by the equation:

$$T_{mn} = \frac{\int_0^\infty t \cdot d(t) \cdot dt}{\int_0^\infty d(t) \cdot dt} \tag{7.1}$$

Details about the fitting procedure are described in appendix B.

7.2.4 Data processing and statistical analysis

The ratio between maximal myocardial flow after and before the PTCA was called the maximal flow ratio (MFR) for the respective ROI and calculated as:

$$MFR = \frac{T_{mn} \text{ before PTCA}}{T_{mn} \text{ after PTCA}} \tag{7.2}$$

Because of the pressure dependency of flow during maximal vasodilation, MFR was corrected for changes in mean arterial pressure in the studies

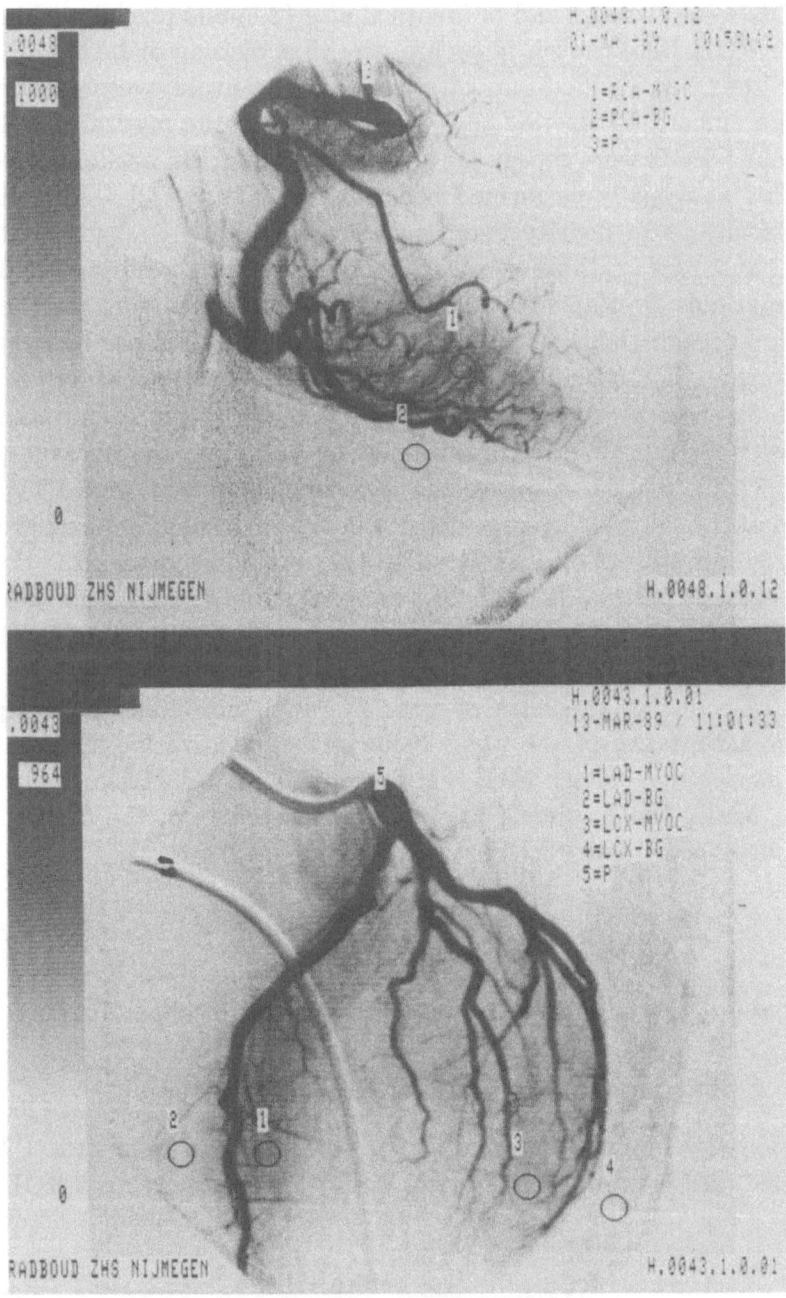

Figure 7.1: *Representative examples of location of regions of interest (ROIs) over the parts of the myocardium supplied by the right coronary artery (top), the left anterior descending artery and the left circumflex artery (bottom), as well as the corresponding background ROIs.*

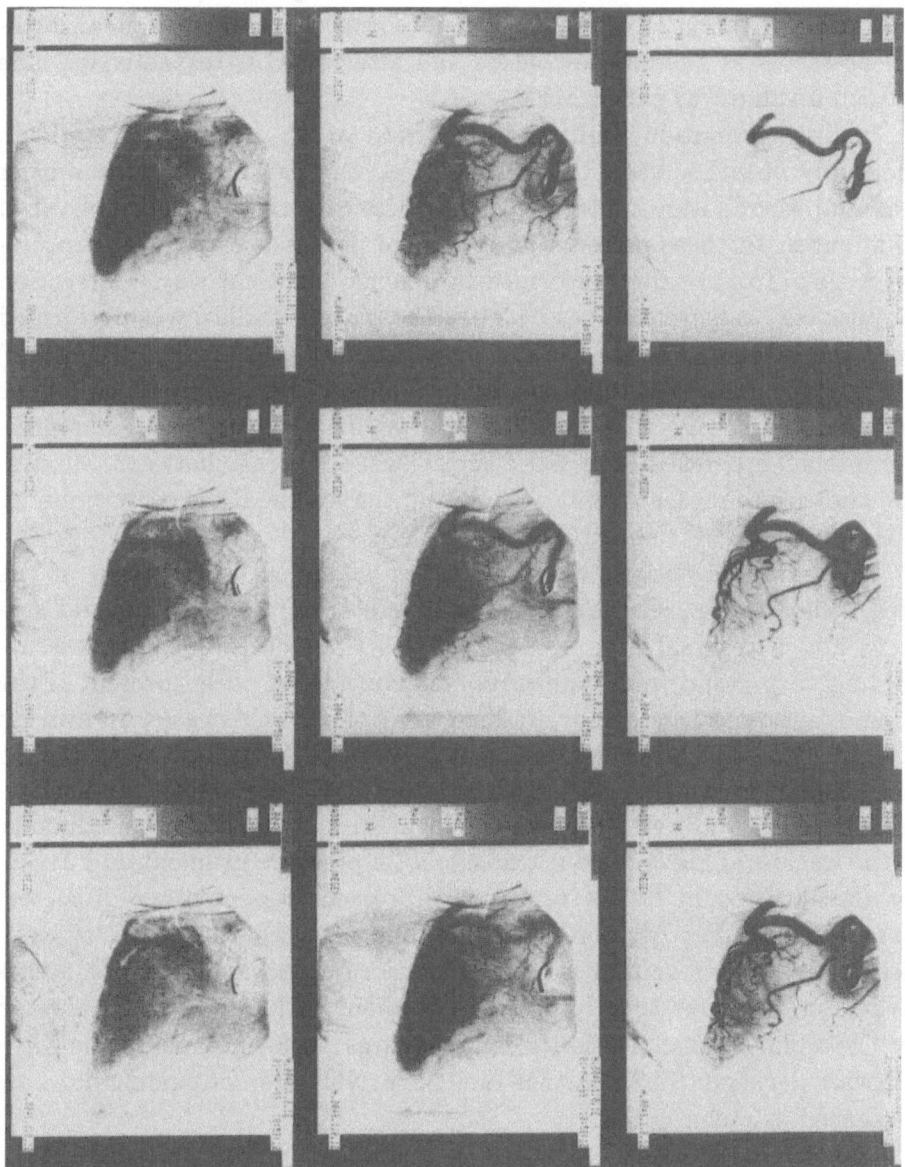

Figure 7.2: *Example of a sequence of mask mode subtracted images of the RCA and its corresponding myocardium in a 68-year-old lady, illustrating filling of the capillary bed by contrast agent and subsequent washout. Contrast injection starts at the 12th heart cycle following start of image acquisition. Image # 11 was chosen as mask. Even on the last image in this series, corresponding with the 26th heart cycle after start of image acquisition, only mild motion artifacts are visible. (From Pijls et al., with permission of the American Heart Association, Inc.)*

before and after PTCA. This was performed by multiplying MFR by the ratio $P_a(1)/P_a(2)$ where $P_a(1)$ and $P_a(2)$ represent the mean arterial pressures at the studies before and after PTCA, respectively. The corrected value was called MFR_c.

In testing reproducibility of calculation of T_{mn} , in 2×10 patients one study of either the LCA or the RCA was performed twice during maximal vasodilation under identical circumstances with an interval of 10 minutes. In these paired studies, image processing and ROI processing were automatically performed in exactly identical way. Correction for possible pressure changes between the paired studies, was performed by multiplying T_{mn} at the second measurement by the ratio $P_a(2)/P_a(1)$ where $P_a(1)$ and $P_a(2)$ represent again the mean arterial pressures at the first and the second of the paired studies, respectively. Linear regression plots were drawn and the correlation coefficients between the first and the second measurement were calculated for the ROIs corresponding with the LAD, LCx and RCA respectively.

Angiographic success of PTCA was defined as a reduction of the area stenosis of at least 20% of the diameter of a nearby normal segment and a residual area stenosis of less than 50% [26]. Success according to pressure measurements was considered to be present if the mean transstenotic pressure gradient after the PTCA was ≤ 15 mm Hg [26, 27]. To determine separation between MFR_c values indicative for successful or unsuccessful PTCA according to ET results, linear discriminant analysis was performed on the logarithmic data. The performance of the angiographic criterion, transstenotic pressure gradient and MFR_c for classification of PTCA results is expressed as percentage of correct classification. Furthermore, the relations between the result of exercise testing and result of the PTCA according to angiographic stenosis reduction, transstenotic pressure gradient or MFR_c, were evaluated by Chi-square tests. Statistical analysis was performed using the SAS-software package (SAS institute Inc, Cary, NC). Hemodynamic data are presented as mean $\pm$ SD.

7.3   Results

7.3.1   Clinical and hemodynamic data

The clinical characteristics of the study population and the data on exercise testing, stenosis severity, pressure gradients, mean transit time before and after PTCA, MFR and MFR$_c$ are tabulated in table 7.1. The mean values ± SD for a number of these parameters are listed in table 7.2. MFR could not be determined in 7 patients: In one patient atrial fibrillation occurred during positioning of the stimulation catheter which was the only complication related to this study. In 3 patients overall image quality was insufficient, due to motion artifacts. In one patient a RCA stenosis could not be passed successfully, in one patient a previously narrowed LCx artery was totally occluded at the time of the PTCA, and in one patient emergency surgery was necessary after a large dissection at the site of a LAD stenosis, which was the only complication related to the PTCA procedure itself in this study population. Transstenotic pressure gradients were not measured in 13 patients because the balloon catheter deemed necessary in these patients by the interventional cardiologist, did not permit pressure measurements.

The frequency of atrial pacing in the study population was 82 ± 10 (range 71 - 107, but always the same in all studies belonging to one patient). Mean arterial pressure was 82 ± 14 mm Hg during the study of the affected artery before PTCA and 77 ± 14 mm Hg thereafter.

PTCA was successful according to eyeball assessment of the stenosis by the interventional cardiologist immediately after the procedure in 36/40 patients and reversal of ET from positive to negative occurred in 30 patients including both patients in whom thallium scintigraphy was performed. After an averaged follow up of 6 months (range 1-13), recurrent angina pectoris occurred in 7 patients, necessitating re-PTCA in 4 of them.

7.3.2 Quality and reproducibility of image acquisition and time-density curves

The average image quality was surprisingly well. Adequate fits to the sampled time-density curves could be obtained in 91% of all studies, the relative error E_r being less than 10%. Some representative examples of images are shown in figure 7.2 and 7.3. Some examples of background corrected time-density curves and the corresponding fits are also presented in figure 7.3. Reproducibility of T_{mn} , obtained from 2 identical studies with an interval of 10 min, was excellent. After correction for the small changes in mean arterial pressure in the paired studies as outlined in the methods section, the correlation coefficients between the first and second measurement were 0.97, 0.95, and 0.95, for the LAD, LCx and

Table 7.1: *Clinical characteristics of the study population and data on exercise testing, densitometric area stenosis severity, transstenotic pressure gradient (ΔP) and mean transit time (T_{mn}) at maximal hyperemia before and after the PTCA (P). MFR_c =maximal flow ratio after correction for pressure changes. $-,+,++$ and $+++$ refer to exercise test results according to Selzer[17]. • indicates that the corresponding value could not be determined (see text).*

| | | | | Exercise Testing | | | |
| | Age | | Affected | ECG-abnorm. | | Exercise Time (s) | |
Patient	(yr)	Gender	Artery	before P	after P	before P	after P
1	69	M	LAD	++	-	2	5
2	64	M	LAD	++	-	5	9
3	40	M	LAD	+	-	7	8
4	68	F	LCX	+++	-	1	5
5	57	F	LAD	++	-	2	6
6	44	M	LAD	-	-	7	9
7	52	M	LAD	-	-	11	12
8	68	F	LAD	+++	-	1	4
9	66	M	LCX	+++	-	5	7
10	60	M	RCA	+++	-	6	11
11	39	M	LAD	+++	-	1	7
12	59	M	RCA	+++	•	6	•
13	55	M	RCA	+	-	4	11
14	54	M	LAD	++	-	2	8
15	68	M	LCX	+	-	7	9
16	41	M	LCX	+	-	6	11
17	57	M	LAD	+	-	4	7
18	69	F	LCX	+	-	4	5
19	44	M	LAD	++	-	8	13
20	67	M	LAD	+++	•	7	•
21	41	M	LAD	++	-	9	12
22	59	F	RCA	++	+	4	4
23	50	M	LCX	-	-	12	12
24	55	F	LAD	+	-	4	5
25	47	M	RCA	-	-	6	10
26	37	M	LAD	+	-	11	14
27	64	M	LAD	+++	-	6	11
28	47	M	LCX	-	-	11	13
29	60	M	LCX	+++	-	9	9
30	40	M	LAD	+++	-	4	13
31	68	F	RCA	+++	-	1	5
32	61	M	LCX	+	-	12	10
33	77	F	LAD	++	+	1	5
34	48	M	LAD	++	-	5	12
35	64	M	RCA	++	-	7	9
36	52	M	RCA	+++	-	6	7
37	55	M	RCA	++	-	9	9
38	61	M	LAD	+	-	7	5
39	54	M	RCA	++	++	8	9
40	47	M	LCX	+	-	12	16

Table 7.1: *continued*

Patient	% stenosis		Transstenotic Δ P (mm Hg)		T_{mn} at max hyperemia (s)		Maximal Flow Ratio	MFR$_c$
	before P	after P	before P	after P	before P	after P		
1	95	75	49	10	•	3.6	•	•
2	84	57	41	10	8.1	2.1	3.9	3.3
3	88	62	58	23	3.5	1.6	2.2	2.0
4	90	16	51	8	10.2	2.4	4.3	4.2
5	91	43	47	14	6.1	1.8	3.4	3.1
6	79	57	•	•	4.5	5.2	1.2	1.2
7	76	45	17	10	4.5	4.0	0.9	0.9
8	89	53	•	•	8.0	3.5	2.3	2.3
9	100	65	•	16	•	3.4	•	•
10	79	40	53	28	7.0	4.4	1.6	1.9
11	84	35	60	38	4.9	1.7	2.9	3.5
12	99	•	•	•	•	•	•	•
13	93	38	•	•	9.7	4.0	2.4	2.4
14	84	21	•	•	4.9	2.2	2.2	1.9
15	90	39	•	•	5.2	2.9	1.8	2.2
16	87	11	42	8	6.5	3.2	2.0	2.0
17	92	42	57	9	8.7	2.9	3.0	3.0
18	77	13	42	15	•	•	•	•
19	67	46	•	•	5.8	2.2	2.6	3.3
20	48	•	•	•	7.2	•	•	•
21	72	46	55	5	5.9	3.1	1.9	1.7
22	71	35	41	16	3.6	3.5	1.0	1.0
23	74	74	•	•	4.5	•	•	•
24	89	30	34	14	7.0	3.1	2.3	3.0
25	90	30	•	•	4.8	3.9	1.2	1.4
26	81	36	36	14	7.5	4.2	1.8	1.9
27	88	41	42	10	10.8	4.1	2.6	2.9
28	86	51	51	11	5.3	2.9	1.8	2.1
29	63	52	41	16	6.0	2.3	2.6	2.2
30	74	9	51	0	5.8	1.7	3.4	3.8
31	90	30	•	•	12.2	5.8	2.2	2.2
32	79	32	•	•	•	•	•	•
33	95	39	30	20	7.6	6.3	1.2	1.3
34	86	19	39	8	8.1	4.7	1.7	1.8
35	92	65	55	9	8.3	7.8	1.1	1.1
36	91	77	•	•	7.3	3.6	2.0	2.0
37	74	60	40	10	8.6	4.9	1.8	2.0
38	77	46	45	9	6.3	2.2	2.9	2.9
39	84	48	52	34	4.9	6.8	0.7	0.8
40	81	26	54	13	5.1	2.3	2.2	2.4

Table 7.2: *Area stenosis severity (determined by quantitative densitometry), transstenotic pressure gradient (ΔP), mean transit time at maximal hyperemia (T_{mn}) and exercise time before and after PTCA (mean $\pm$ SD).*

	Pre-PTCA	Post-PTCA	n
% Area stenosis	83 ± 10	42 ± 18	38
Transstenotic ΔP (mm Hg)	45 ± 10	14 ± 9	27
T_{mn} at max hyperemia (s)	6.9 ± 2.1	3.4 ± 1.4	33
Exercise time (s)	350 ± 191	520 ± 76	38

Table 7.3: *Relations between maximal flow ratio after correction for pressure changes (MFR_c), angiographic success, and trans-stenotic pressure gradient as measured 5 minutes after the last balloon inflation (Δ P), and presence or absence of reversal of exercise test (ET) result. (+ indicates positive ET; - indicates negative ET) Angiographic success was defined as $\geq$ 20% area stenosis reduction and residual area stenosis <50%, calculated by quantitative coronary arteriography.*

MFR_c / E.T	> 1.6	< 1.6
+ → -	25	1
+ → + / - → -	1	6

E.T	ANGIO. SUCC	ANGIO. UNSUCC
+ → -	21	9
+ → + / - → -	4	4

ΔP / E.T	< 15 mm Hg	> 15 mm Hg
+ → -	17	5
+ → + / - → -	2	3

Table 7.4: *Mean transit time (s) at maximal coronary and myocardial hyperemia corresponding with stenotic vessels before and after PTCA and with normal control vessels (mean ± SD). LAD = Left Anterior Descending Artery; LCx = Left Circumflex Artery; RCA = Right Coronary Artery; Number of data: see figure 7.4.*

	stenotic artery		control artery
	before PTCA	after PTCA	
LAD	6.6 ± 1.8	3.0 ± 1.1	3.2 ± 0.8
LCx	6.3 ± 2.0	2.9 ± 0.4	3.3 ± 0.6
RCA	7.7 ± 2.7	4.7 ± 1.5	4.6 ± 1.0

RCA respectively. Reproducibilty will be discussed more extensively in chapter 8.

7.3.3 Relation between MFR and exercise tests results

Mean transit time was 6.9 ± 2.1 s before and 3.4 ± 1.4 s after PTCA. After correction for pressure changes as indicated above, this corresponded with a relative increase in maximal myocardial perfusion of $224 \pm 149\%$ (range 80 - 420%). If only those patients with a successful PTCA according to ET results were considered, the pressure-corrected increase in maximal flow was $249 \pm 73\%$. MFR_c was correlated to presence or absence of reversal of ET result from positive to negative. By linear discriminant analysis, maximal separation was yielded by a MFR_c value of 1.6. Therefore MFR_c of > 1.6 or < 1.6 was chosen for further evaluation (table 7.3).

MFR_c was > 1.6 in 26 patients. In 25 of these patients, a positive ET 1-2 days before the intervention became negative 7 days thereafter. In the remaining patient (#28) a severe stenosis in a posterolateral branch of the LCx artery had been present 24 days before PTCA and at that

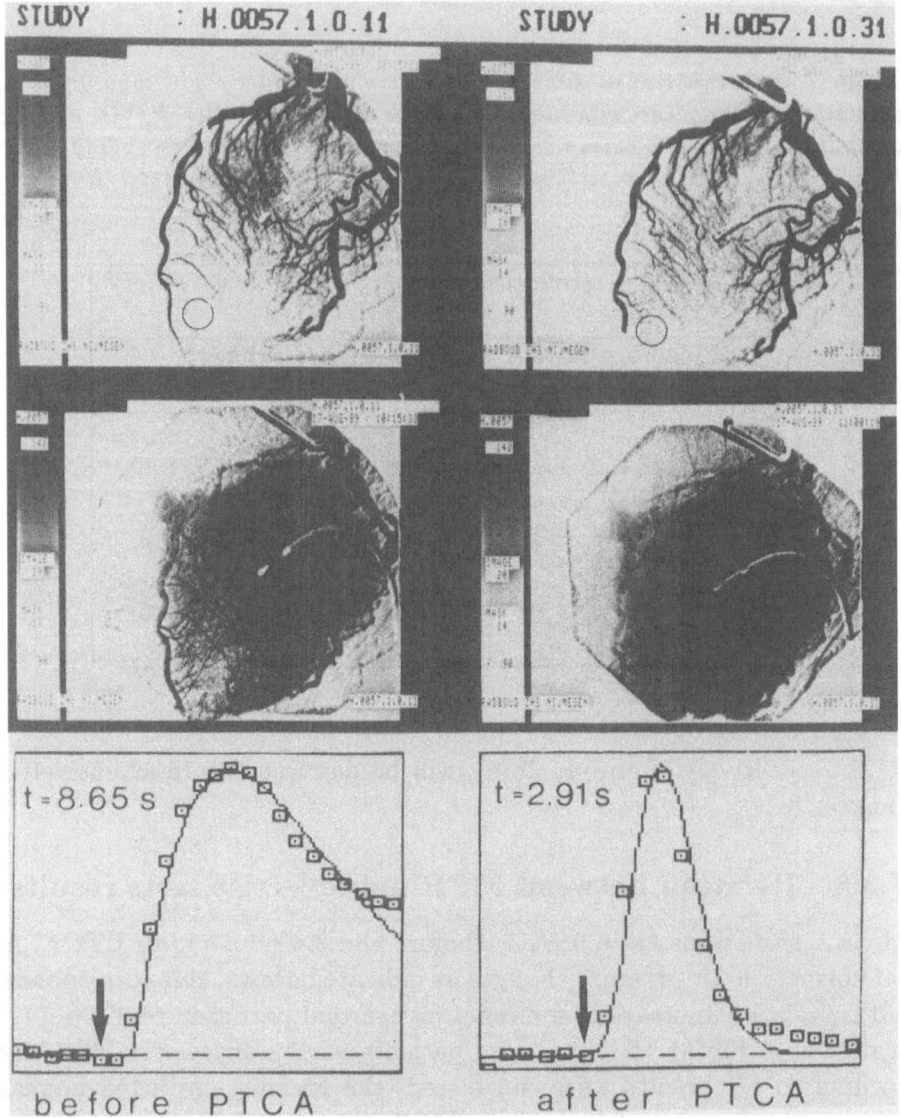

Figure 7.3: *Left anterior descending artery of a 57-year-old male before PTCA (left series) and after PTCA (right series) and the corresponding background corrected time-density curves. The functional effect of the LAD-stenosis is pronounced and these images enable clear detection of the perfusion defect. After PTCA, coronary anatomy has moderately improved but a dissection is present at the site of balloon inflation. Nevertheless, rapid and complete filling of the apex occurs this time. Time density curves, derived from a region of interest over the apex (circle) are presented in the lower part of the figure. Mean transit time was 8.7 s before and 2.9 s after PTCA, corresponding with an increase in maximal flow of 300%. The arrows indicate the moment of start of the contrast injection.*

(From Pijls et al., with permission of the American Heart Association, Inc.)

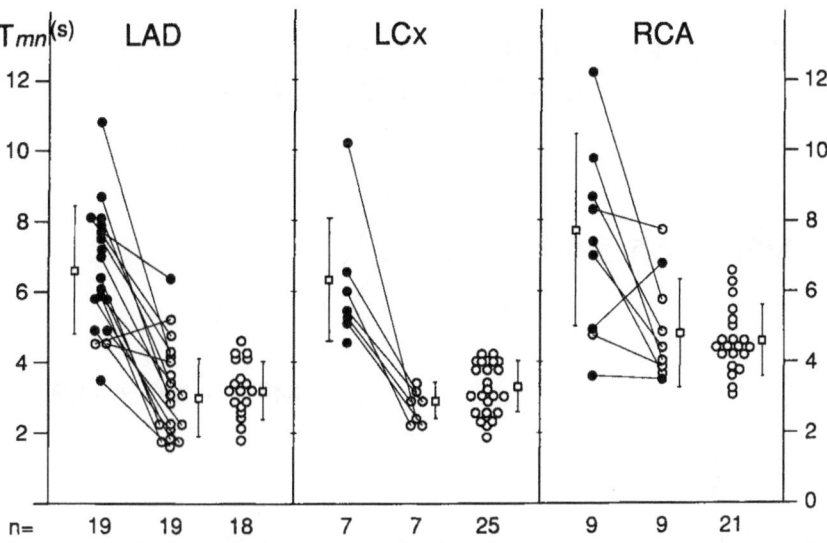

Figure 7.4: *Values for mean transit time (s) at maximal myocardial hyperemia belonging to stenotic vessels before (B) and after (A) successful PTCA and to normal control vessels (C). LAD = left anterior descending artery; LCx = left circumflex artery; RCA = right coronary artery. The closed points correspond with a positive exercise test and the open points with a negative exercise test. The mean value ± SD is indicated in the figure. (From Pijls et al., with permission of the American Heart Association, Inc.)*

time this patient had severe anginal complaints and a positive ET. After prolonged nocturnal pain 2 weeks before the PTCA, anginal complaints had disappeared. The ET 24 hours prior to PTCA was negative and remained so after successful dilation of the LCx stenosis with a MFR_c of 2.1. This course suggests that a small infarction had occurred at the time of prolonged nocturnal pain and that PTCA had been unnecessary.

MFR_c was < 1.6 in 7 patients and in 6 of these 7 patients no reversal of ET result was observed: In 3 of these patients (#6, 7, 25) anginal complaints and a positive ET had been present 2- 6 weeks earlier and a significant stenosis was found at that time. Two days before the PTCA, however, a maximal ET was performed without anginal complaints or ECG abnormalities. At PTCA, the stenosis was still present and apparently unchanged in all of these patients. T_{mn} , however, was already

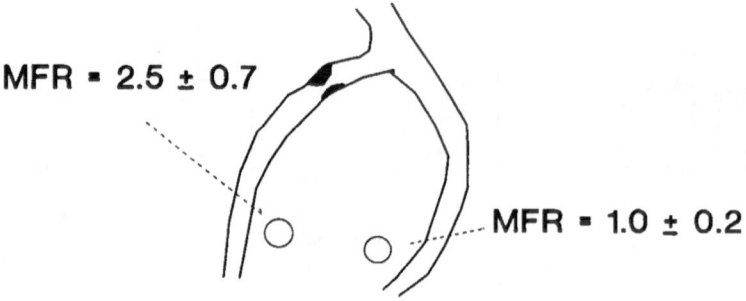

ONE STENOTIC BRANCH OF LCA ⎤ N ▪ 30
ONE NORMAL BRANCH OF LCA ⎦

MFR ▪ 2.5 ± 0.7

MFR ▪ 1.0 ± 0.2

Figure 7.5: *Maximal Flow Ratio for the dilated branche of the left coronary artery and for the normal branche which served as a control vessel (mean value ± SD).*

rather short before PTCA and remained so thereafter, resulting in a MFR_c of 1.2, 0.9 and 1.4 respectively. This strongly suggests that, between the time of acceptance and actual performance of the PTCA, the functional significance of the stenosis had diminished in these patients and the necessity of these 3 PTCAs can be considered doubtful. In the remaining 3 patients without reversal of ET result (#22, 33, 39) , PTCA was not successful and a positive ET remained positive. In all of these patients T_{mn} remained almost unchanged, resulting in a MFR_c of 1.0, 1.3 and 0.8 respectively. In only one patient (#35) a previously positive ET became negative after PTCA despite absence of decrease of T_{mn} over the myocardium of the dilated artery. No explanation is present in this case.

In table 7.3, it can be seen that MFR_c more or less than 1.6, determined from studies immediately before and 15 min after PTCA, is highly predictive for functional success or failure as indicated by ET (correct classification in 94%, $\chi^2 = 21.9, p < 0.001$). If, on the contrary, on-line evaluation of the PTCA result was based upon angiographic criteria or upon measurement of transstenotic pressure gradient, the relation with ET result was significantly worse (correct classification in 66% and 74%

respectively, $\chi^2 = 1.20$ and 2.64 respectively).

7.3.4 Comparison of T_{mn} belonging to apparently normal arteries and to stenotic arteries before and after successful PTCA

In this population of 40 patients with single vessel disease, 64 values of T_{mn} of apparently normal coronary arteries could be obtained. The 16 missing values are due to the reasons mentioned in one of the former sections ($n = 9$), to presence of a rudimental RCA ($n = 2$) and to presence of wall irregularities $> 20\%$ as judged by an independent reviewer ($n = 5$).

A definite range of time could be distinguished for T_{mn} at maximal hyperemia corresponding with these apparently normal vessels (figure 7.4 and table 7.4). These values were compared with measurements of T_{mn} of the affected artery before and after PTCA. Before PTCA, T_{mn} is long and covers a wide range as expected. After successful PTCA, T_{mn} returns to the 'normal' range. Some overlap between normal and affected arteries is present in case of the RCA.

In 25/30 patients in whom a stenotic LAD or LCx artery was dilated, T_{mn} of the normal branch of the left coronary artery could be compared before and after PTCA. MFR$_c$ for these control vessels was 1.0 ± 0.2 (figure 7.5).

At last, the ratio (T_{mn} diseased branch of the LCA) / (T_{mn} normal branch of the LCA) was calculated in this group. This ratio is not dependent on pressure and decreased from 1.9 ± 0.3 before PTCA to 0.9 ± 0.3 after PTCA.

7.4 Discussion

The videodensitometric approach for flow measurement as used in this clinical study, was very similar to the method validated in animal experiments before [15]. In that validation study it was proved, that comparison of maximal myocardial flow between situations with different degrees of stenosis can be performed accurately by calculating ratios of mean transit time.

In this clinical study, after extensive training to hold breath and using synchronous X-ray pulses, image quality was so good that passage of contrast agent through the myocardium could be studied long enough to allow reliable determination of T_{mn} in about 90% of the patients. Reproducibility of T_{mn} in paired studies under identical circumstances was excellent. Therefore, it can be concluded that this videodensitometric approach is applicable in clinical practice, at least in stable patients, and the first aim of this study has been achieved by that.

A difference between the previously mentioned experimental study and this clinical study is the different method to induce maximal hyperemia. In the validation study, continuous infusion of dipyridamole was applied for this purpose [15]. For practical reasons, such as short time of activity, intracoronary papaverine was used in the clinical study. It has been proved by former investigators that from approximately 25 to 60 seconds after i.c. administration of 8-12 mg of papaverine, maximal dilation of the myocardial vascular bed is achieved [28, 29]. Therefore we assumed that during acquisition of the time-density curve, the vascular volume remained maximal and constant, whereas flow was not influenced by contrast injection.

In this clinical study, exercise testing 24-48 hours before and 7-10 days after the PTCA was the method of choice for non- invasive functional evaluation of the result of the procedure. Because in all patients the combination of anginal complaints NYHA class III, a positive ET and proved single vessel disease had been present less than 6 weeks before the PTCA, exercise testing can discriminate accurately between presence or absence of (residual) ischemia in this particular group of patients [30, 31]. Moreover, because of the presence of just single vessel disease, it is justified to assume that ischemia, if present at exercise testing, is actually caused by the affected artery [30]. Therefore, ET results could be used in this study as the gold standard for PTCA success. MFR_c , angiographic result, and final transstenotic pressure gradient were correlated to this gold standard.

Because exercise testing after the PTCA was performed several days after the flow measurements, changes in coronary anatomy and physiology could have occurred in the meantime. The 94% agreement between MFR_c and ET seems to be high in this respect. If, however, PTCA result in this study was judged by classical anatomic criteria, a previously positive ET remained positive despite an angiographically successful intervention in 3 patients (#22,33,39), leading to a functional restenosis rate of 12% within one week which is in accordance with current literature [32, 33].

One may speculate if this finding merely reflects the hypothesis that insufficient increase in flow after PTCA is a better predictor for restenosis than coronary anatomy.

The approach used in this study for calculation of flow is only valid in situations of maximal vasodilation to guarantee constant vascular volume. It should be emphasized that no information about resting flow can be obtained and therefore no coronary flow reserve can be calculated. This approach, however, offers the possibility to compare maximal myocardial flow before and after an appropriate intervention, such as angioplasty in this study but possibly also long-lasting lipid lowering therapy. Unlike coronary flow reserve, this maximal flow ratio is independent of resting flow which is in turn influenced by heart rate, left ventricular hypertrophy, previous infarction in other segments, prolonged ischemia and the PTCA procedure itself [1, 12, 16], [34] - [39]. At maximal vasodilation, flow is only dependent on pressure which can easily be measured and corrected for as was done in this study. In fact, MFR_c as defined in this study can be considered as the improvement of relative coronary flow reserve as recently defined by Gould et al [40]. It should be realized in this context that anginal complaints in the majority of patients are due to inadequate maximal flow. Therefore, increase in maximal flow is a clinically relevant parameter and is expected to reflect improved exercise tolerance.

In the practice of interventional cardiology, parameters for on- line evaluation of the result of the intervention are essential. Because T_{mn} can be calculated within minutes after image acquisition and decrease of this value correlates well with the functional result of the PTCA, determination of MFR_c can be used for this purpose.

Despite their limitations, some other methods have been used for on-line evaluation of the PTCA until now, such as assessment of angiographic stenosis severity or measurement of trans-stenotic pressure gradients [26, 27, 41, 42]. Therefore we also investigated the relation between these on-line parameters and ET results 7-10 days after the procedure. Both parameters were significantly less reliable than the use of MFR_c.

In most former videodensitometric approaches, flow has been represented by contrast density divided by a certain time parameter such as appearance time [6, 7, 8, 43]. Because contrast density, expressed in arbitrary units, is dependent on many factors not related to flow, and differs more than thousand percents between different patients, it has been regarded as impossible to indicate normal values in these studies.

Because in the present study merely a time parameter is used as an index of flow, it makes sense to look if a range of normal values for T_{mn} at maximal hyperemia does exist. Most of the patients in this study provided 2 apparently normal coronary arteries and indeed a definite range for T_{mn} of these normal vessels during maximal hyperemia could be distinguished. This means that, also in diagnostic catheterization, one single determination of T_{mn} at maximal coronary hyperemia may provide useful information about the functional significance of a coronary artery stenosis.

In this study, after successful PTCA according to exercise testing, T_{mn} returned to the 'normal' range except in one case (#35) (figure 7.4). In previous studies using digital radiography for evaluation of CFR improvement after PTCA, it was observed that CFR immediately after the intervention did not return to normal [43, 44]. It has been hypothesized that this phenomenon could be caused by the fact that resting flow after PTCA would still be elevated due to prolonged ischemia and to the procedure itself [14, 43, 44]. Our results are in favour of this explanation because T_{mn} at maximal flow in the dilated vessel was not longer than T_{mn} at maximal flow in apparently normal coronary arteries. Furthermore, in those 30 patients with one diseased and one normal branch of the left coronary artery, the ratio (T_{mn} diseased artery) / (T_{mn} normal artery) decreased from 1.9 ± 0.3 before PTCA to 0.9 ± 0.3 after PTCA, which gives further support to that explanation. This last observation also suggests that the ratio between T_{mn} of a stenotic and of a normal branch can help to assess the functional significance of the stenosis. Finally, it was observed in this group that the MFR_c of normal control vessels was 1.0 ± 0.2 which argues for the intrinsic correctness of this method (figure 7.5).

7.5   Limitations

For the time being, the approach suggested in this study only provides an index for the maximal flow achievable for a certain vascular bed prior to and following an intervention. Although a certain range of normal values could be distinguished in this special group of patients, it is still to early to judge about its value for the diagnostic catheterization. More data about normal coronary arteries are necessary. It should be remarked in this context that inadequate MFR can either mean that the

PTCA failed or that the situation before the PTCA was already (nearly) normal and that, in fact, PTCA had not been necessary as was probably the case in 3 of our patients (#6, 7, 25). This ambiguity between an unsuccessful intervention and an anatomically successful intervention in a distribution without baseline flow abnormality, could restrict the clinical usefulness of this approach. As can been observed in figure 7.4, however, knowledge of normal values for T_{mn} during maximal hyperemia can help to discriminate between these possibilities. In case of the LAD and LCx arteries, an excellent partition between pathologic and normal values is present. In case of the RCA there is some overlap. In case of a stenosis in one branch of the LCA, also the ratio (T_{mn} diseased branch)/(T_{mn} normal branch) can be helpful in this respect.

A further limitation is, that acquisition of well interpretable time-density curves is highly dependent on sufficient image quality. In this study adequate image acquisition both before and after PTCA was possible in about 90% of all patients but one can doubt on this point in case of emergency situations where no chance for previous training to hold breath is present. In that case, motion artifacts serious enough to interfere with reliable image processing, may be present more often.

The population in this study consisted of a selected homogeneous group of patients with single vessel disease. Although from a theoretical point of view there is no reason why this approach would not be valid in multivessel disease, some caution is warranted in extrapolation of these results to other groups of patients. The reason to confine this study to patients with single vessel disease, was to be sure of an unambiguous functional test to decide about success or failure of the intervention. As explained above, exercise testing could be used for this purpose in this particular group of patients. In multivessel disease, on the contrary, a positive ET even if combined with thallium scintigraphy, is hard to relate to one particular stenosis [16, 18].

Another factor which may restrict the clinical value of the MFR, is the presence of collateral circulation, excluded in this study. In that case, transport of contrast agent injected into the vessel itself can be slowed down by collateral blood supply. This also holds true for patients with bypass grafts in whom the native vessel is not completely occluded.

Next, it is necessary that overprojection of the myocardium supplied by the analyzed artery can be avoided while nevertheless its thickness in the chosen projection should be large enough to ensure sufficient staining after contrast injection. This can be hard to obtain for diagonal and intermediate branches of the LAD artery and for posterolateral branches of the LCx artery.

At last it should be remarked that, in case of serial lesions within one vessel, T_{mn} at maximal hyperemia for the supplied vascular bed tells something about the summed effect of all abnormalities and nothing about the significance of the individual lesions. This might, however, also be an advantage, e.g. in studies to the effects of long-lasting lipid lowering therapy, if one is interested in the functional status of an artery and not in individual lesions.

Despite these limitations, this study shows that comparison of maximal flow before and after PTCA is possible in at least a large part of patients and enables reliable, on-line evaluation of the functional improvement achieved by the intervention.

References

[1] White C W, Wright C B, Doty D B, Hiratza L F, Eastham C L, Harrison D G, and Marcus M L. Does visual interpretation of the coronary arteriogram predict the physiological importance of a coronary stenosis? *N Engl J Med*, 310:819–824, 1984.

[2] Nissen S E, Elion J L, Booth D C, Evans J, and DeMaria A N. Value and limitations of computer analysis of digital subtraction angiography in the assessment of coronary flow reserve. *Circulation*, 73:562–571, 1986.

[3] Kirkeeide R L, Gould K L, and Parsel L. Assessment of coronary stenoses by myocardial perfusion imaging during pharmacologic coronary vasodilation. VIII. Validation of coronary flow reserve as a single integrated functional measure of stenosis severity reflecting all its geometric dimensions. *J Am Coll Cardiol*, 7:103–113, 1986.

[4] Vogel R, LeFree M, Bates E, O'Neill W, Foster R, Kirlin P, Smith D, and Pitt B. Application of digital techniques to selective coronary arteriography: use of myocardial appearance time to measure coronary flow reserve. *Am Heart J*, 107:153–164, 1984.

[5] Vogel R A, Bates E R, O'Neill W W, Aueron F M, Meier B, and Gruentzig A R. Coronary flow reserve measured during cardiac catheterization. *Arch Intern Med*, 144:1773–1776, 1984.

[6] Hodgson J M, Legrand V, Bates E R, Mancini G B J, Aueron F M, O'Neill W W, Simon S B, Beauman G J, LeFree M T, and Vogel R A. Validation in dogs of a rapid digital angiographic technique to measure relative coronary blood flow during routine cardiac catheterization. *Am J Cardiol*, 55:188–193, 1985.

[7] Vogel R A. Radiographic assessment of coronary blood flow parameters. *Circulation*, 72:460–465, 1985.

[8] Bates E R, Aueron F M, Legrand V, LeFree M T, Mancini G B J, Hodgson J M, and Vogel R A. Comparative long-term effects of coronary artery bypass graft surgery and percutaneous transluminal coronary angioplasty on regional coronary flow reserve. *Circulation*, 72:833–839, 1985.

[9] Cusma J T, Toggart E J, Folts J D, Peppler W W, Hagiandreou N J, Lee C S, and Mistretta C A. Digital subtraction imaging of coronary flow reserve. *Circulation*, 75:461–472, 1987.

[10] Ikeda H, Koga Y, Utsu F, and Toshima H. Quantitative evaluation of regional myocardial blood flow by videodensitometric analysis of digital subtraction coronary arteriography in humans. *J Am Coll Cardiol*, 8:809–816, 1986.

[11] Nishimura R A, Rogers P J, Holmes D R, Gehring D G, and Bove A A. Assessment of myocardial perfusion by videodensitometry in the canine model. *J Am Coll Cardiol*, 9:891–897, 1987.

[12] Hoffman J I E. Maximal coronary flow and the concept of coronary vascular reserve. *Circulation*, 70:153–159, 1984.

[13] Vogel R A. Assessing stenosis significance by coronary arteriography: are the best variables good enough? *J Am Coll Cardiol*, 12:692–693, 1988.

[14] Nissen S E and Gurley J C. Assessment of the functional significance of coronary stenoses. is digital angiography the answer? *Circulation*, 81:1431–1435, 1990.

[15] Pijls N H J, Uijen G J H, Hoevelaken A, Arts T, Aengevaeren W R M, Bos H S, Fast J H, Van Leeuwen K L, and Van der Werf T. Mean transit time for the assessment of myocardial perfusion by videodensitometry. *Circulation*, 81:1331–1340, 1990.

[16] Gould K L. Identifying and measuring severity of coronary artery stenosis. Quantitative coronary arteriography and positron emission tomography. *Circulation*, 78:237–245, 1988.

[17] Selzer A, Cohn K, and Goldschlager N. On the interpretation of the exercise test. *Circulation*, 58:193–195, 1978.

[18] Rigo P, Bailey I K, Griffith L S C, Pitt B, Burow R D, Wagner H N, and Becker L C. Value and limitations of segmental analysis of stress thallium myocardial imaging for localization of coronary artery disease. *Circulation*, 61:973–981, 1980.

[19] Van der Werf T, Heethaar R M, Stegehuis H, and Meijler F L. The concept of apparent cardiac arrest as a prerequisite for coronary digital subtraction angiography. *J Am Coll Cardiol*, 4:239–244, 1984.

[20] Katritsis D, Lythall D A, Cooper I C, Crowther A, and Webb-Peploe M. Assessment of coronary angioplasty: comparison of visual assessment, hand-help caliper measurement and automated digital quantitation. *Cathet Cardiovasc Diagn*, 15:237–242, 1988.

[21] Bevington P R. *Data reduction and error analysis for the physical sciences*, pages 204–246. McGraw-Hill, New York, 1969.

[22] Press W H, Flannery B P, Tenkolsky S A, and Vettering W T. *Numerical recipes. The art of scientific computing*, pages 523–528. Cambridge University Press, Cambridge, 1987.

[23] Uijen G H J, Pijls N H J, and Van der Werf T. The accuracy of densitometric time parameters in the analysis of myocardial perfusion. In *Computers in Cardiology 1988*, pages 215–218. IEEE Computer Society, Washington DC, 1989.

[24] Zierler K L. *Circulation times and the theory of indicator dilution methods for determining blood flow and volume*, pages 585–615. American Physiological Society, Washington DC, 1962.

[25] Rutishauser W, Simon H, Stucky J P, Schad N, Noseda G, and Wellauer J. Evaluation of roentgen cinedensitometry for flow measurement in models and in the intact circulation. *Circulation*, 36:951–963, 1967.

[26] Kent K M, Bentivoglio L G, Block P C, Cowley M J, Dorros G, Gosselin A J, Gruentzig A R, Myler R K, Simpson J, Stertzer S H, Williams D O, Fisher L, Gillepsie M J, Detre K, Kelsey S, Mullin S M, and Mock M B. Percutaneous transluminal coronary angioplasty: report from the Registry of the National Heart Lung and Blood Institute. *Am J Cardiol*, 49:2011–2020, 1982.

[27] MacIsaac H C, Knudtson M L, Robinson V J, and Manyari D E. Is the residual translesional pressure gradient useful to predict regional myocardial perfusion after percutaneous transluminal coronary angioplasty? *Am Heart J*, 117:783–790, 1989.

[28] Wilson R F, Laughlin D E, Ackell P H, Chilian W M, Holida M D, Hartley C J, Armstrong M L, Marcus M L, and White C W. Transluminal subselective measurement of coronary artery blood flow velocity and vasodilator reserve in man. *Circulation*, 72:82–92, 1985.

[29] Zijlstra F, Serruys P W, and Hugenholtz P G. Papaverine: the ideal coronary vasodilator for investigating coronary flow reserve? A study of timing, magnitude, reproducibility and safety of the coronary hyperemic response after intracoronary papaverine. *Cathet Cardiov Diagn*, 12:298–299, 1986.

[30] Hamilton G W, Trobaugh G B, Ritchie J L, Gould K L, DeRouen A, and Williams D L. Myocardial imaging with [201]thallium: An analysis of clinical usefulness based on bayes' theorem. *Semin Nucl Med*, 8:358–364, 1978.

[31] Melin J A, Piret L J, Vanbutsele R J M, Rousseau M F, Cosyns J, Brasseur L A, Beckers C, and Detry J M R. Diagnostic value of exercise electrocardiography and thallium myocardial scintigraphy in patients without previous myocardial infarction: a Bayesian approach. *Circulation*, 63:1019–1024, 1981.

[32] Nobuyoshi M, Kimura T, Nosaka H, Mioka S, Keno K, Yohoi H, Hamasaki N, Horiuchi H, and Ohishi H. Restenosis after successful percutaneous transluminal coronary angioplasty: serial angiographic follow-up of 299 patients. *J Am Coll Cardiol*, 12:616–623, 1988.

[33] Serruys P W, Rensing B F, Luyten H E, Hermans W R M, and Beatt K J. *Restenosis following coronary angioplasty*, pages 79–115. Hogreve & Huber Publishers, Goettingen, 1990.

[34] Marcus M, Wright C, Doty D, Eastham C, Laughlin D, Krumm P, Fastenow C, and Brody M. Measurements of coronary velocity and reactive hyperemia in the coronary circulation of humans. *Circ Res*, 49:877–891, 1981.

[35] O'Neill W W, Walton J A, Bates E R, Colfer H T, Aueron F M, LeFree M T, Pitt B, and Vogel R A. Criteria for successful coronary angioplasty as assessed by alterations in coronary vasodilatory reserve. *J Am Coll Cardiol*, 3:1382–1390, 1984.

[36] Klein L W, Agarwal J B, Schneider R M, Hermann G, Weintraub W S, and Helfant R H. Effects of previous myocardial infarction on measurements of reactive hyperemia and the coronary vascular reserve. *J Am Coll Cardiol*, 8:357–363, 1986.

[37] Klocke F J. Measurements of coronary flow reserve: defining pathophysiology versus making decisions about patient care. *Circulation*, 76:1183–1189, 1987.

[38] Serruys P W, Juilliere Y, Zijlstra F, Beatt K J, De Feyter P J, Suryapranata H, Van den Brand M, and Roelandt J. Coronary blood flow velocity during percutaneous transluminal coronary angioplasty as a guide for assessment of the functional result. *Am J Cardiol*, 61:253–259, 1988.

[39] Vogel R A and Mancini G B J. Assessment of coronary flow and myocardial perfusion with digital radiography. In G B J Mancini, editor, *Clinical applications of cardiac digital angiography*, pages 281–290. Raven Press, New York, 1988.

[40] Gould K L, Kirkeeide R L, and Buchi M. Coronary flow reserve as a physiologic measure of stenosis severity. *J Am Coll Cardiol*, 15:459–474, 1990.

[41] Chokshi S K, Meyers S, and Abi-Mansour P. Percutaneous transluminal coronary angioplasty: ten years' experience. *Prog Cardiovasc Dis*, 30:147–210, 1987.

[42] Rothman M T, Baim D S, Simpson J B, and Harrison D C. Coronary hemodynamics during PTCA. *Am J Cardiol*, 49:1615–1622, 1982.

[43] Zijlstra F, Den Boer A, Reiber J H C, Van Es G A, Lubsen J, and Serruys P W. Assessment of immediate and long-term results of percutaneous transluminal coronary angioplasty. *Circulation*, 78:15–24, 1988.

[44] Zijlstra F, Reiber J C, Juilliere Y, and Serruys P W. Normalizaiton of coronary flow reserve by percutaneous transluminal coronary angioplasty. *Am J Cardiol*, 61:55–60, 1988.

Chapter 8

Reproducibility of Mean Transit Time for Maximal Myocardial Flow Assessment

8.1 Introduction

After injection of contrast agent into a coronary artery, time density curves (TDCs) over myocardial regions of interest (ROIs) can be obtained, using ECG-triggered digital radiography. These TDCs resemble indicator dilution curves and contain useful information about myocardial perfusion [1, 2, 3]. In the previous chapters, it has been shown that an excellent correlation exists between inverse mean transit time (T_{mn}), derived from these curves under maximal hyperemic conditions and maximal myocardial blood flow [4, 5]. The purpose of the present study was to investigate reproducibility of T_{mn} determination at maximal hyperemia in man.

In determining reproducibility of time parameters obtained by videodensitometry, reproducibility of image acquisition and of image processing should be distinguished. In former studies several investigators demonstrated that, given a certain series of images, intra-observer and inter-observer variability in the different steps of image processing, in particular the placement of ROIs and calculation of time parameters from the TDCs, are very small, even if ROIs are of irregular shape and drawn by hand [6, 7, 8, 9, 10]. In the approach as used in this study and described more extensively in some previous papers, all ROIs are circular and of identical size and are placed automatically in the same place within all sequences of images (studies) within one individual [4, 5].

Therefore, no concern is present about variations in image processing. Because, however, a large part of the TDC has to be known to calculate T_{mn} and because the shape of especially the descending part of the TDC can change considerably with changes in image quality, T_{mn} can be expected to be subject to variability in image acquisition more than any other time parameter [4, 7]. Nevertheless, in animal validation studies reproducible determination of T_{mn}, obtained from sequential series of images, turned out to be possible in dogs with percentual differences of about 5% [4]. These studies, however, were performed under anesthesia and with the use of muscle relaxing drugs. In this study we tested reproducibility of T_{mn} determination at maximal hyperemia in sequential studies in conscious man during routine cardiac catheterization.

8.2   Methods

8.2.1   Study protocol and image acquisition

Twenty patients, accepted for elective coronary arteriography, were seen at the outpatient's department 2 days before the actual investigation. The purpose of the study was explained to them and this was followed by extensive breathholding training at maximal inspiration, using a nose clamp and laying in the same position as foreseen for the catheterization. All patients were trained to hold breath during at least 20 seconds and careful attention was paid to avoid motion of head, neck, shoulders, and thorax during the holding of breath. Patients were asked to repeat this training at home at night and also the next day after admission to the hospital. At the time of coronary arteriography, two additional ECG-triggered, digital studies at maximal hyperemia were performed of either the left coronary artery (LCA, $n = 10$) or the right coronary artery (RCA, $n = 10$) under identical circumstances with an interval of 5-10 minutes. For both studies, 6 ml Iohexol-350 (Nycomed, Oslo, Norway) was injected at a speed of 4 ml/s, using a power injector (Sybron Angiomat 300). Contrast injections started 30 seconds after intracoronary administration of papaverine, 8 mg in the RCA or 12 mg in the LCA, to assure maximal dilation of the myocardial vascular bed during image acquisition. One image was sampled per heart cycle, just before the onset of the QRS-complex. Studies of the RCA were performed in the 30° right anterior oblique projection and studies of the LCA in the 60° left anterior oblique projection, in which the myocardium supplied

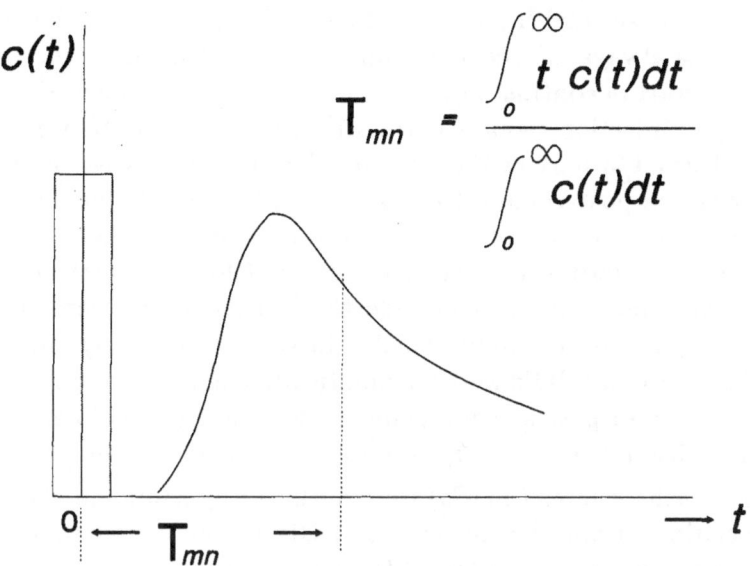

Figure 8.1: *Temporal relations and definition of time t = 0. Contrast injection is considered as a block pulse with a width of 1.5 s. Therefore, t=0 is defined as the moment 0.75 s after start of contrast injection, which is registered in a ROI at the tip of the coronary catheter. Mean transit time (T_{mn}) of the contrast agent from the injection site to the myocardial ROI is defined according to theory.*

by the left anterior descending (LAD) and the left circumflex (LCx) artery are well separated. The paced heart rate was slightly higher than the intrinsic heart rate and identical in the paired studies, while arterial pressure was continuously recorded during image acquisition. Care was taken to avoid changes in the patient's position between the paired studies and all imaging variables, such as table position, image intensifier, etc, were frozen during the 5-10 min interval.

8.2.2 Image processing and processing of TDCs

Image acquisition and processing were performed using a Siemens Bicor X-ray equipment in connection with a Siemens Digitron 3 image processor (Siemens AG, Erlangen, FRG). Images were digitized in a 512×512 matrix with 1024 density levels. In the first of the paired studies, a region of interest (ROI) was chosen over the tip of the coronary catheter to record start of contrast injection. Because the duration of the contrast injection was always 1.5 seconds, time = 0 was defined as the moment 0.75 s after start of contrast injection, being the mean transit time of the block shaped injection signal (figure 8.1). Myocardial ROIs were chosen over the distal 1/3 part of the antero-apical region in case of the LAD artery, over the posterolateral region at the level of the posteromedian papillary muscle in case of the LCx artery and over the mid portion of the posterior septum in case of the RCA. Close to these myocardial ROIs, background ROIs just outside the heart contour were chosen to detect changes in background density. In the second study, all myocardial and background ROIs were automatically placed in exactly the same position on the display screen. Only a few times, manual correction of the ROI position was necessary due to some motion of the patient.

Time density curves (TDCs) were obtained by sampling the average pixel densities within the myocardial ROIs in the consecutive images. These curves were corrected by subtraction of the sampled average background densities. A gamma function was fitted to the remaining data in analogy to former studies. The quality of the fit was tested by calculating the relative error E_r. Only if this error was less than 10% the curve was accepted. T_{mn} was calculated from the fit function according to theory [4, 11, 12]. Details about curve fitting and processing are described in Appendix B.

8.2.3 Data processing and statistical analysis

Values for T_{mn}, obtained from the paired studies, were compared by calculating the ratio of the difference between both measurements and the first measurement (relative difference) both before and after correction for possible changes in mean arterial pressure between both studies. Correction for pressure changes between the first and the second of the paired studies, was performed by multiplying T_{mn} at the second measurement with the ratio $P_a(2))/P_a(1)$ where $P_a(1)$ and $P_a(2)$ are the mean arterial pressures during the respective series of image acquisition. To facilitate visual interpretation of the data, also the relation between both measurements was plotted and linear regression analysis was performed. The data were evaluated for all arteries together and for the LAD, LCx, and RCA separately. Results are expressed as mean ± SD.

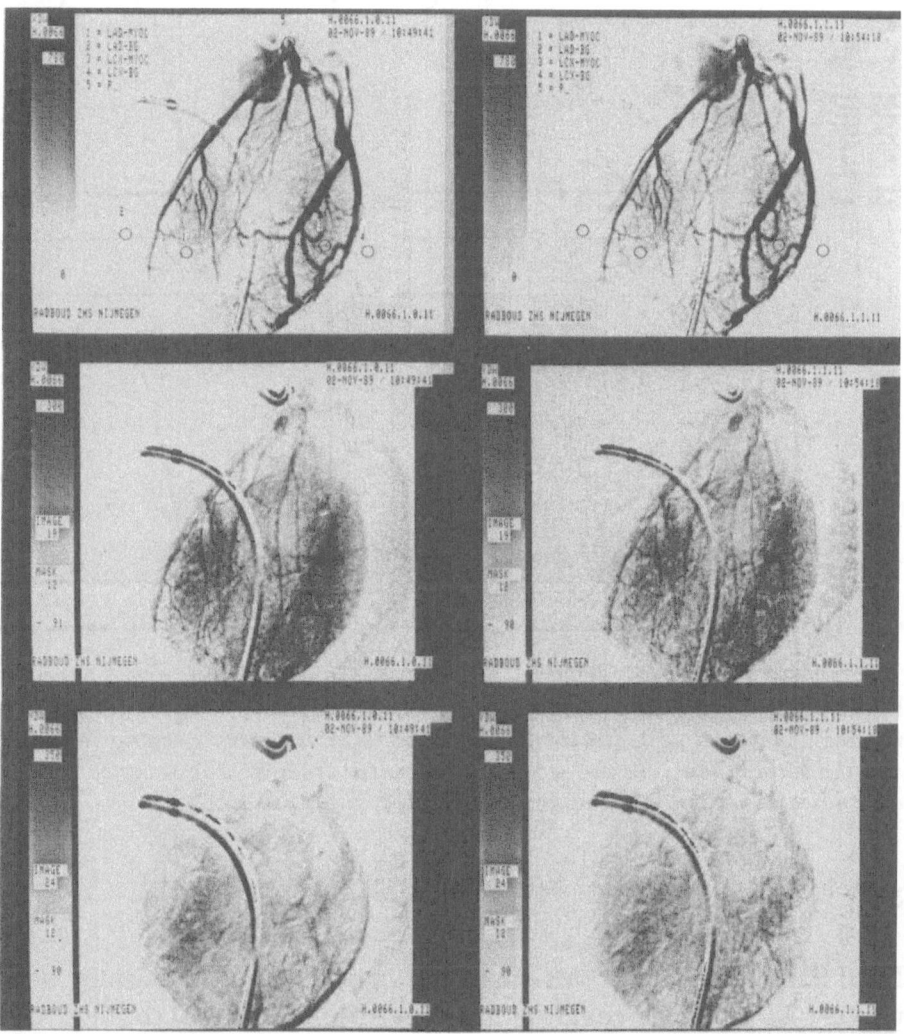

Figure 8.2: *Representative example of paired studies of the left coronary artery in one patient. The left hand side of the figure belongs to the first series of images, the right hand side to the second series, made 10 minutes later. From top to bottom, the 3rd, 7th, and 12th image after start of contrast injection are shown, representing the coronary phase, the myocardial wash-in, and the myocardial wash-out phase of the contrast passage at maximal hyperemia.*

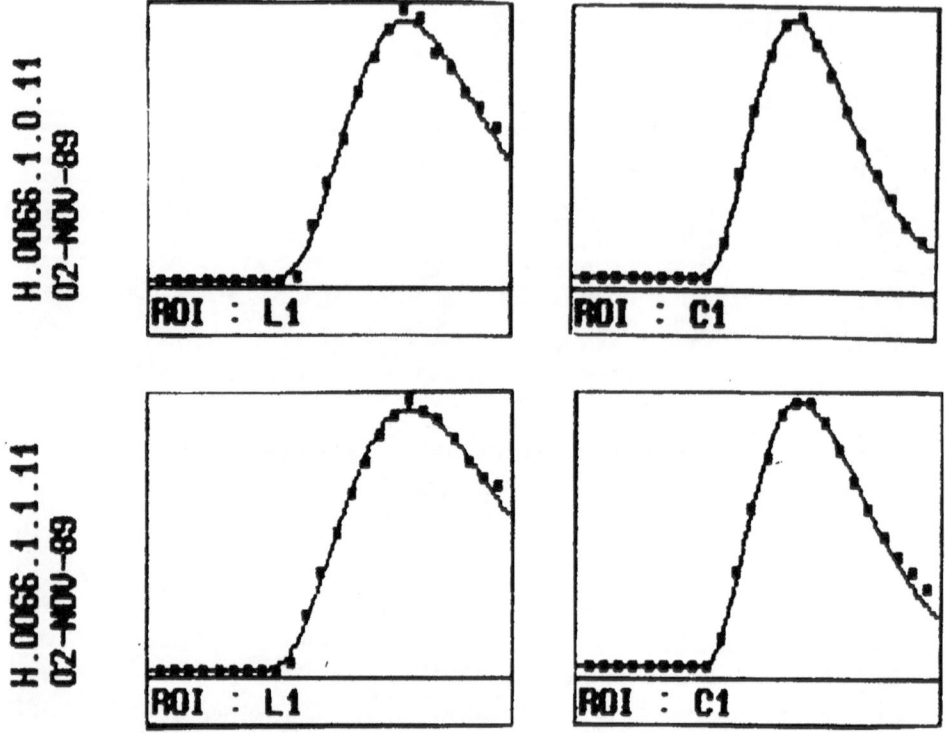

Figure 8.3: *Background corrected time-density curves, corresponding with the regions of interest as indicated in figure 8.2. The top panels belong to the first and the bottom panels to the second of the paired studies. The sampled densities are indicated by the bold squares and the best fit by the line.*

8.3   Results

In all but one patient in this study, image quality was sufficiently well to provide TDCs which could be fitted by the gammafit according to the condition as described in the methods. Some representative examples of images and curves of the paired studies in one patient are presented in figure 8.2 and 8.3.

Mean arterial pressure was 82 ± 14 mm Hg in the first study and 83 ± 13 mm Hg in the second one. The difference in mean arterial pressure between both studies was 1 ± 5 mm Hg. In table 8.1, age and gender, T_{mn} at maximal hyperemia in the first and in the second study, and the relative difference between these observations before and

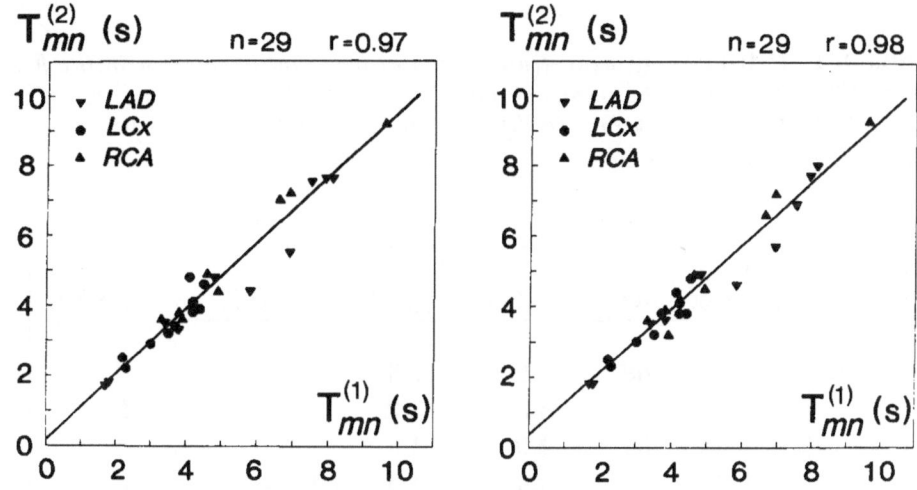

Figure 8.4: *Relation between mean transit time at maximal hyperemia at the first ($T_{mn}^{(1)}$) and the second ($T_{mn}^{(2)}$) measurement, before (left) and after (right) correction for pressure changes. The line represents the line of identity. Values, derived from the myocardium of the left anterior descending, left circumflex, and right coronary artery are indicated by the inverse triangles, circles, and upright triangles respectively.*

after correction for pressure changes. As can be seen, the differences are almost always small for all 3 coronary arteries. The morphology of the vessels covered the complete range between normal and subtotal stenosis.

The mean values of the relative differences between the first and the second measurement of T_{mn}, as well as their absolute values before and after pressure correction, are shown in table 8.2 for the respective arteries and for the collected data. The average values for the coefficients of variation are also presented in table 8.2. In figure 8.4 the paired measurements are plotted both before and after correction for pressure changes. The correlation coefficients between both values for T_{mn} are 0.97, 0.91, and 0.98 for the LAD, LCx, and RCA respectively before pressure correction and 0.97, 0.95, and 0.95 thereafter, the slope always being close to 1.0, and the interception close to 0.

Table 8.1: *Patient data, mean transit time at maximal hyperemia in the first study ($T_{mn}(1)$) and in the second study ($T_{mn}(2)$) and the relative difference between both observations before ($\Delta\%$) and after ($(\Delta\%)_c$) correction for pressure changes.* • = *missing value*

	#	sex	age	$T_{mn}(1)$	$T_{mn}(2)$	$\Delta\%$		$(\Delta\%)_c$	
LAD	1	F	68	7.9	7.6	-	4	-	3
	2	M	59	3.8	3.3	-	13	-	9
	3	M	54	4.9	4.9		0	+	4
	4	M	41	3.4	3.5	+	3	+	3
	5	M	41	5.8	4.4	-	24	-	18
	6	M	50	1.8	1.8		0		0
	7	F	55	6.9	5.5	-	20	-	17
	8	M	37	7.5	7.5		0	-	8
	9	M	40	1.7	1.7		0	+	6
	10	M	48	8.1	7.6	-	6	-	1
LCx	1	F	68	4.2	4.1	-	2	-	2
	2	M	59	3.8	3.3	-	13	-	9
	3	M	54	3.0	2.9	-	3		0
	4	M	41	3.5	3.2	-	9	-	9
	5	M	41	2.3	2.2	-	4		0
	6	M	50	4.4	3.9	-	11	-	13
	7	F	55	4.5	4.6	+	2	+	7
	8	M	37	4.1	4.8	+	17	+	7
	9	M	40	2.2	2.5	+	14	+	18
	10	M	48	3.7	3.4	-	8	-	3
RCA	11	M	55	9.6	9.2	-	4	-	3
	12	M	47	4.9	4.4	-	10	-	8
	13	M	50	3.3	3.6	+	9	+	9
	14	M	52	•	•		•		•
	15	M	48	6.9	7.2	+	4	+	4
	16	M	44	3.9	3.6	-	8	-	18
	17	M	51	3.8	3.8		0	+	3
	18	F	65	6.6	7.0	+	6		0
	19	M	54	4.2	4.0	-	5		0
	20	M	42	4.6	4.9	+	7	+	7

Table 8.2: *Mean ± S.D. of the relative differences (Δ%), their absolute values before (|Δ%|) and after (|(Δ%)$_c$|) correction for pressure changes for the left anterior descending (LAD), left circumflex (LCx), and right coronary artery (RCA), and for the collected data.*

	Δ%	|Δ%|	|(Δ%)$_c$|
LAD (n=10)	-6 ± 9	7 ± 9	7 ± 7
LCx (n=10)	-2 ± 10	8 ± 5	6 ± 3
RCA (n=9)	0 ± 7	5 ± 3	4 ± 2
All (n=29)	-3 ± 9	7 ± 6	5 ± 5

8.4   Discussion

For reliable determination of T_{mn} by videodensitometry, a large part of the TDC, including its descending part, has to be known. For this reason determination of this time parameter is dependent on constant and high quality of image acquisition [1, 2, 3, 4, 7]. Therefore, demonstration of reproducible determination of T_{mn} from sequential series of images acquired under identical circumstances, is mandatory before this time parameter can be used for maximal flow assessment in man. In this study, excellent and reproducible image quality proved to be possible in this group of elective patients, and by locating the ROIs in exactly the same way in the paired studies, variability in image processing was excluded. Mean transit time was calculated from the gammafit to the sampled data, and only if the fit fulfilled the preset criterion of an E_r of < 10%, this fit was accepted, which was the case in all but one patient. In this way reproducible calculation of T_{mn} proved to be possible.

As shown in table 8.1, in almost all patients the changes between the first and second measurement were small. Because all studies were performed at maximal vasodilation, flow has become dependent on pressure only and therefore a correction was made if changes in mean arterial pressure occurred between both studies [13]. After this pressure correction, the differences were even smaller.

It should be remarked that maximal efforts were made to exercise to hold breath and to avoid motion artifacts in the study population. Therefore, this approach seems to be less suitable for emergency patients in whom there is a lack of time for training and instructions. In our approach, training and instructions take about 30 minutes and are mandatory to obtain an image quality good enough to provide reliable time density curves.

From this study it can be concluded that determination of T_{mn} at maximal hyperemia can be performed in a reproducible way in patients during cardiac catheterization. Because changes in T_{mn} at maximal hyperemia are inversely related to changes in the maximal myocardial perfusion achievable for a certain vascular bed [4], a reliable method is provided to compare maximal flow under different circumstances within one individual patient. Therefore, by this method a useful means to evaluate the functional effect of mechanical or medical interventions is at disposal.

References

[1] Rutishauser W, Simon H, Stucky J P, Schad N, Noseda G, and Wellauer J. Evaluation of roentgen cinedensitometry for flow measurement in models and in the intact circulation. *Circulation*, 36:951–963, 1967.

[2] Rutishauser W, Bussmann W D, Noseda G, Meier W, and Wellauer J. Blood flow measurement through single coronary arteries by roentgen densitometry. part I: A comparison of flow measured by a radiologic technique applicable in the intact organism and by electromagnetic flowmeter. *Am J Roentgenol*, 109:12–20, 1970.

[3] Rutishauser W, Noseda G, Bussman W D, and Preter B. Blood flow measurement through single coronary arteries by roentgen densitometry. Part II: Right coronary artery flow in conscious man. *Am J Roentgenol*, 109:21–24, 1970.

[4] Pijls N H J, Uijen G J H, Hoevelaken A, Arts T, Aengevaeren W R M, Bos H S, Fast J H, Van Leeuwen K L, and Van der Werf T. Mean transit time for the assessment of myocardial perfusion by videodensitometry. *Circulation*, 81:1331–1340, 1990.

[5] Pijls N H J, Uijen G J H, Hoevelaken A, Pijnenburg T, Van Leeuwen K, Fast J H, Bos J S, Aengevaeren W R M, and Van der Werf T. Mean transit time for videodensitometric assessment of myocardial perfusion and the concept of maximal flow ratio: A validation study in the intact dog and a pilot study in man. *Int J Cardiac Imag*, 5:191–202, 1990.

[6] Hodgson J M, Legrand V, Bates E R, Mancini G B J, Aueron F M, O'Neill W W, Simon S B, Beauman G J, LeFree M T, and Vogel R A. Validation in dogs of a rapid digital angiographic technique to measure relative coronary blood flow during routine cardiac catheterization. *Am J Cardiol*, 55:188–193, 1985.

[7] Vogel R A. Radiographic assessment of coronary blood flow parameters. *Circulation*, 72:460–465, 1985.

[8] Zijlstra F, Den Boer A, Reiber J H C, Van Es G A, Lubsen J, and Serruys P W. Assessment of immediate and long-term results of percutaneous transluminal coronary angioplasty. *Circulation*, 78:15–24, 1988.

[9] Vogel R A and Mancini G B J. Assessment of coronary flow and myocardial perfusion with digital radiography. In G B J Mancini, editor, *Clinical applications of cardiac digital angiography*, pages 281–290. Raven Press, New York, 1988.

[10] Whiting J S, Drury J K, Pfaff J M, Chang B L, Eigler N L, Meerbaum S, Corday E, Nivatpumin T, Forrester J S, and Swan H J C. Digital angiographic measurement of radiographic contrast material kinetics for estimation of myocardial perfusion. *Circulation*, 73:789–798, 1986.

[11] Zierler K L. *Circulation times and the theory of indicator dilution methods for determining blood flow and volume*, pages 585–615. American Physiological Society, Washington DC, 1962.

[12] Uijen G H J, Pijls N H J, and Van der Werf T. The accuracy of densitometric time parameters in the analysis of myocardial perfusion. In *Computers in Cardiology 1988*, pages 215–218. IEEE Computer Society, Washington DC, 1989.

[13] Gould K L, Kirkeeide R L, and Buchi M. Coronary flow reserve as a physiologic measure of stenosis severity. *J Am Coll Cardiol*, 15:459–474, 1990.

Chapter 9

General Discussion

9.1 Discussion

The heart is the engine that powers life and the coronary circulation is the lifeline to transport blood to the myocardium. This blood contains oxygen and substrate to maintain the metabolic processes which keep the heart beating.

Atherosclerotic narrowing of the coronary arteries, leading to impairment of myocardial blood supply, constitutes the most frequent cause of mortality in the western world. To estimate and understand the pathophysiologic significance of such a narrowing, knowledge about its influence on blood flow is of paramount importance. The relevance of endeavours to assess flow, therefore, is indisputable [1, 2, 3, 4].

In this book, efforts are described to obtain information about flow by analyzing the myocardial passage of contrast agent, injected into a coronary artery at cardiac catheterization. A major advantage of such an approach is, that no additional investigations are necessary. More, previously hidden, information is derived from the same data. Besides conventional catheterization data, insight into the physiologic significance of the lesion, i.e. its impeding effect on flow, is obtained.

The background theory for this method is provided by the classical indicator dilution theory. Almost 25 years ago, Rutishauser suggested that myocardial flow measurement should be possible by studying contrast passage [5, 6, 7]. Application of these concepts in conscious man during cardiac catheterization, however, has been hampered by many problems. Unproven assumptions and violations of physiologic principles could not be avoided until recently [3, 4]. As extensively discussed in chapter 4, 6, and 7, expressing flow as the ratio of vascular volume and mean transit time (T_{mn}), requires absence of influence of the indicator (contrast agent) on flow, a constant vascular volume, linearity between contrast density and contrast concentration, and reliable determination of T_{mn}. In the current approach, the first three conditions are fulfilled by merely working at maximal coronary and myocardial hyperemia, and the latter one by a significant improvement of image quality (and therefore time-density curve quality) which will be discussed below.

Merely working under maximal hyperemic conditions means that no information about resting flow can be obtained. As discussed in chapter 6 and 7, however, maximal flow is the clinically most relevant index of the maximal performance of the myocardium. Therefore, we believe that this restriction is not a disadvantage.

The correctness and accuracy of the method described in this book, was demonstrated in an animal validation study [8]. Because in this animal model flow was not influenced by contrast injection and vascular volume remained constant, an ideal opportunity was present to elucidate basic physiologic principles and to study the value of former hypotheses in this field, which state that appearance time of contrast agent could be used as a reliable time parameter and maximal contrast intensity as an index of volume. The shortcomings of these previous approaches could be clearly demonstrated, as well as the superiority of T_{mn} to assess flow. Reflecting upon the value of contrast density for flow assessment, we have become suspicious anyhow: in many of our studies we have learned that it is illusory to assume that the same amount of contrast agent will enter a particular branch of the coronary tree at different injections, unless subselective injections are performed. This also explains why normal ranges could never be distinguished in former approaches, which are, unlike the current method, dependent on contrast density.

In the clinical studies, reliable and reproducible application of our approach proved to be possible in conscious patients undergoing elective catheterization or coronary angioplasty (PTCA). Changes in maximal flow as indicated by T_{mn}, showed an excellent correlation with the functional result of an intervention. Useful ranges of values of T_{mn}, corresponding with normal coronary arteries, could be established [9, 10, 11].

9.2   Conclusions

The main conclusions from the invesigations described in this book can be summarized as follows:

A. Assessment of maximal myocardial blood flow can be performed reliably by videodensitometry, using mean transit time as a parameter of flow. This can be done strictly in accordance with the principles of the indicator dilution theory.

B. In this way a reliable method is provided to evaluate changes in maximal flow as a result of an intervention. This evaluation can be performed on-line. In case of a PTCA, it can be used for decision making during the course of the procedure. Increase in maximal flow, achievable by the myocardium supplied by the dilated artery, is the best correlate of functional improvement of the patient.

C. Ranges of normal values of mean transit time at maximal hyperemia can be discriminated. Therefore, this method can be used during routine diagnostic cardiac catheterization to obtain information about the functional significance of a stenosis in a coronary artery by one single contrast injection at maximal hyperemia.

D. After successful PTCA, maximal flow through the dilated lesion immediately returns to the normal range.

9.3   Limitations

A number of limitations still do exist. Most of these have already been discussed in detail in the former chapters.

   A practical limitation is that this approach is dependent on a high image quality. The studies in humans were performed in elective patients who could be well instructed before. In over 90% of these patients sufficient image quality could be achieved. In emergency patients, where no opportunity for previous training to hold breath is present, a higher dropout rate may be expected. A minor practical point is that the catheterization procedure will be prolonged by 20-30 minutes.

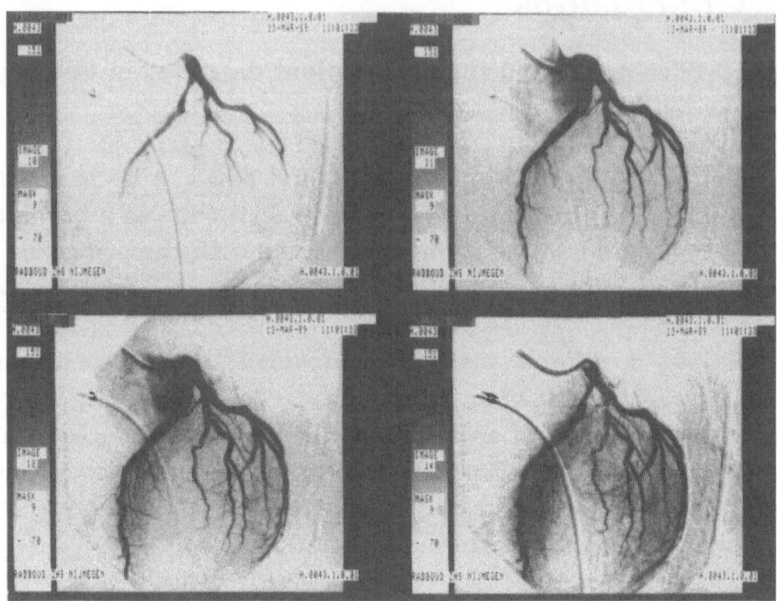

Figure 9.1: *A: Left coronary arteriogram of a 43-year-old male after successful PTCA of the LAD artery. The parts of the myocardium supplied by the LAD and LCx arteries are equally well filled.*

Next, some methodological limitations do exist. So far, the validity of our concept has been demonstrated in patients with single vessel disease. Studies in more complex anatomic states are necessary. As discussed in chapter 7, multivessel disease, left ventricular hypertrophy, previous infarction, rapid heart rate and other pathologic states are not expected to constitute real limitations: all these factors confound only or predominantly determination of resting flow and have no significant influence on maximal flow. Collateral circulation, for the time being, will remain a problem because only flow through the native vessel is measured.

At last, one fundamental question remains unsolved, i.e. the relation between perfusion and contractile function. Proceeding from an anatomic interpretation of coronary arterial lesions to measurement of their impeding effect on blood flow, is one important step. Does, however, sufficient flow always correlate with sufficient contractile capacity? Is the contractile dysfunction shortly after myocardial infarction in the

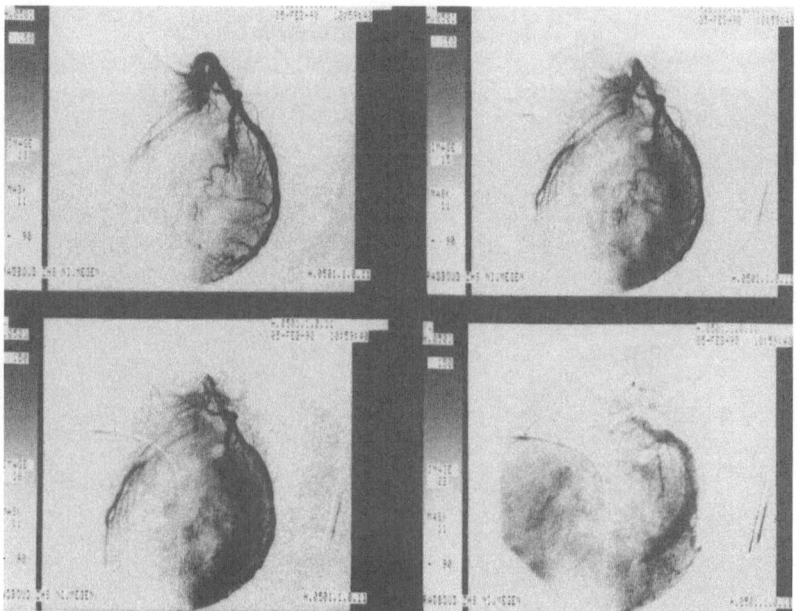

Figure 9.1: *B: Left coronary arteriogram of a 55-year-old male, 3 weeks after an extensive anterior wall myocardial infarction. The perfusion defect of the antero-septal regions of the myocardium can be well appreciated.*

presence of an open or re-opened artery caused by remaining capillary hypoperfusion (no-reflow phenomenon) or is the myocardium itself well perfused and the perfusion-contraction coupling disturbed? A similar problem is present in case of hibernating or stunned myocardium and in situations in which weaning from the extracorporal circulation after cardiac surgery is troublesome. Although the quest for the answers to these questions is beyond the scope of this book, the present method may contribute to solve these clinical problems [3].

9.4 Spin-off and Present Applications

The continuous endeavours to improve the quality of the subtracted images were not an aim in itself, but only served as a means to enable reliable calculation of mean transit time. Nevertheless, also the value of classical angiograms increases with better image quality and during the last years we have been surprised numerous times by images, showing

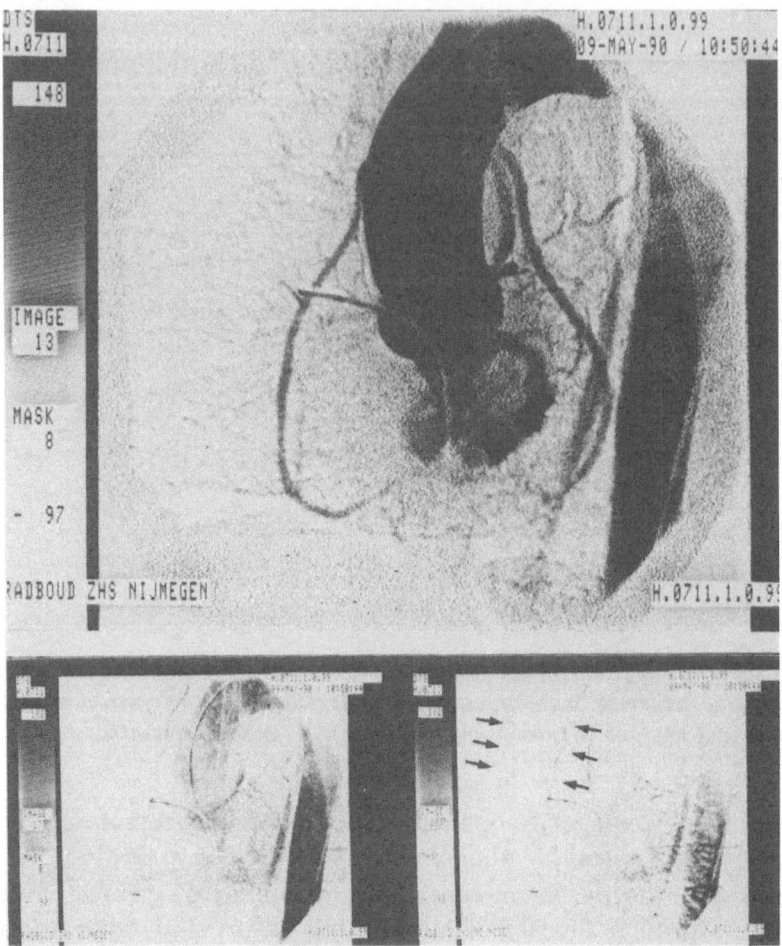

Figure 9.2:. *Nonselective contrast injection into the ascending aorta of a patient who had bypass surgery 3 years previously. Patency of the grafts can easily be judged. In the latter filling phase, patency of both mammarian arteries can be judged as well.*

certain aspects of coronary arteries and the myocardium in more detail than before.This can be elucidating and useful in clinical practice.

Areas of hypoperfusion can be clearly recognized and collateral circulation easily detected. Without selective contrast injections, patency of bypasses can be evaluated. In the previous chapters, a number of examples of this image quality has already been presented (figure 7.1, 7.2,

7.3, and 8.2). Some additional illustrations are presented in figure 9.1 and 9.2.

At the moment, this flow measurement technique is applied in some controlled clinical trials on the influence of long-lasting lipid lowering therapy on the coronary arterial system. Cardiac catheterization is performed in these trials at the beginning and the end of a 2-year treatment period, which is considered as the intervention. In this kind of studies, sophisticated methods have been developed to score progression or regression of coronary atherosclerosis. A final judgement, however, often remains hazardous: especially in the case of multiple lesions within one vessel, plaques may either show regression or progression, which makes it hard to estimate the net effect of the therapy. If, on the contrary, one studies the maximally achievable flow to the distal myocardium supplied by such a vessel, one integral measure is obtained for the summed effect of all lesions which reflects improvement or impairment at the end of the study period.

Other present studies are directed to define ranges of hyperemic T_{mn} under different pathologic conditions and to unravel the complex relation between myocardial perfusion disturbance and abnormalities of contractile state. From these studies we hope to acquire more insight into the sequence of coronary anatomy, myocardial perfusion, and contractile function.

References

[1] White C W, Wright C B, Doty D B, Hiratza L F, Eastham C L, Harrison D G, and Marcus M L. Does visual interpretation of the coronary arteriogram predict the physiological importance of a coronary stenosis? *N Engl J Med*, 310:819–824, 1984.

[2] Klocke F J. Measurements of coronary flow reserve: defining pathophysiology versus making decisions about patient care. *Circulation*, 76:1183–1189, 1987.

[3] Nissen S E and Gurley J C. Assessment of the functional significance of coronary stenoses. is digital angiography the answer? *Circulation*, 81:1431–1435, 1990.

[4] Gould K L. Functional measures of coronary stenosis severity at cardiac catheterization. *J Am Coll Cardiol*, 16:198–199, 1990.

[5] Rutishauser W, Simon H, Stucky J P, Schad N, Noseda G, and Wellauer J. Evaluation of roentgen cinedensitometry for flow measurement in models and in the intact circulation. *Circulation*, 36:951–963, 1967.

[6] Rutishauser W, Bussmann W D, Noseda G, Meier W, and Wellauer J. Blood flow measurement through single coronary arteries by roentgen densitometry. part I: A comparison of flow measured by a radiologic technique applicable in the intact organism and by electromagnetic flowmeter. *Am J Roentgenol*, 109:12–20, 1970.

[7] Rutishauser W, Noseda G, Bussman W D, and Preter B. Blood flow measurement through single coronary arteries by roentgen densitometry. Part II: Right coronary artery flow in conscious man. *Am J Roentgenol*, 109:21–24, 1970.

[8] Pijls N H J, Uijen G J H, Hoevelaken A, Arts T, Aengevaeren W R M, Bos H S, Fast J H, Van Leeuwen K L, and Van der Werf T. Mean transit time for the assessment of myocardial perfusion by videodensitometry. *Circulation*, 81:1331–1340, 1990.

[9] Pijls N H J, Uijen G J H, Hoevelaken A, Pijnenburg T, Van Leeuwen K, Fast J H, Bos J S, Aengevaeren W R M, and Van der Werf T. Mean transit time for videodensitometric assessment of myocardial perfusion and the concept of maximal flow ratio: A validation study in the intact dog and a pilot study in man. *Int J Cardiac Imag*, 5:191–202, 1990.

[10] Pijls N H J, Uijen G J H Aengevaeren W R M, Hoevelaken A, Pijnenburg T, Van Leeuwen K, and Van der Werf T:. The concept of maximal flow ratio for immediate evaluation of Percutaneous Transluminal Coronary Angiography result by videodensitometry. *Circulation*, 83:854–865, 1991.

[11] Pijls N H J, Uijen G J H, Pijnenburg T, Van Leeuwen K, Aengevaeren W R M, Barth J D, Den Arend J, Hoevelaken A, and Van der Werf T:. Reproducibility of mean transit time for maximal myocardial flow assessment by videodensitometry. *Intern J Cardiac Imag*, 6:101–108, 1991.

Appendix A

Is Nonionic Isotonic Iohexol the Contrast Agent of Choice for Quantitative Myocardial Videodensitometry?

In this appendix, a study is described to find an inert indicator, i.e. a contrast agent with minimal influence on coronary flow and other hemodynamic parameters. This study preceded the other investigations described in this book. Although progress was made, no indicator could be found which was sufficiently inert but still enabled adequate image acquisition. Nevertheless, this study is described here because it contains useful background information about contrast agents and imaging procedures and ultimately led to the idea to assess maximal flow rather than coronary flow reserve.

A.1   Introduction

Image subtraction was introduced into radiologic practice over 50 years ago by Ziedzes des Plantes with the purpose to enhance image quality of films with poor definition [1]. In recent years, the same principle has been applied in cardiology, facilitated by the possibility to digitize X-ray images [2]. This resulted in excellent information about the patho-anatomy of coronary vessels. Moreover, by studying contrast passage through myocardial regions of interest, time-density curves could be obtained providing pathophysiologic information concerning myocardial perfusion. Time parameters are defined according to the mathematical theory [3]. In the density analysis the signal on the vertical axis is, after logarithmic transformation, proportional to the product of iodine concentration and the thickness of the vascular compartment containing the contrast, encomprised in the region of interest.

These time-density curves, however, cannot be treated like classical dye dilution curves to calculate flow because of uncertainty about a number of points. In the first place, the exact quantity of iodine, injected into the coronary artery, is unknown because of loss of the contrast agent into the ascending aorta. Secondly, the distribution of the injected quantity over the different myocardial areas is unknown, especially in case of stenoses. Thirdly, the vascular fraction of wall thickness is unknown.

Moreover, comparison of relative myocardial perfusion in different areas or under different circumstances can only be achieved by calculating relative differences in mean transit time. It is important to realize that this time parameter is related to flow but also to vascular volume between injection site and measuring site. Since flow equals volume divided by mean transit time, this last parameter may be compared from one situation to another only if vascular volume remains constant.

In assessment of time-density curves, however, all currently used contrast agents induce a considerable hyperemic response up to 400% during registration of the time-density curve itself [4, 5, 6, 7]. This means that, although some qualitative information can be obtained from these curves, quantitative analysis is hampered seriously.

One possible solution to enable analysis of time-density curves according to indicator dilution theory, is to find a contrast agent with no or negligible reactive hyperemia due to contrast injection.

Injection of currently used contrast agents is believed to cause reactive hypermia by several mechanisms: primary vasodilation by a direct vascular effect due to hyperosmolality and the chemotoxic effect on the red blood cell membrane and secondary vasodilation by alteration of myocardial oxygen demand as a result of changes in heart rate, arterial pressure, or inotropic state.

In search for an ideal contrast medium, the first step was to look for an isotonic agent and attention was drawn to one of the newer nonionic contrast media namely iohexol-140 (Omnipaque-140^R) being the only commercially available isotonic contrast agent at the time of this study. The characteristics of this agent are presented in table A.1.

To exclude the influence of heart rate on oxygen demand, a strictly regular rate was necessary. Although for iohexol no significant influence

Table A.1: *Physical and chemical properties of the studied contrast agents and of blood.*

	iohexol 140	diatrizoate 30%	blood
iodine content (mg/ml)	140	146	-
osmolality (mosm/kg)	290	710	280-300
viscosity at 37° C (mPa.s)	1.5	1.4	3.2-4.0
sodium content (mmol/l)	0	63	138-144

on heart rate has been described, atrial pacing would be preferable for comparison with other, rate influencing contrast agents. Cardiac pacing is necessary anyhow if digital subtraction is used.

According to some investigators, the positive inotropic effect of non-ionic contrast agents is related to changes in cation content of myocardial extracellular fluid and coronary sinus blood, suggesting a Ca^{++} dependency of this effect [5]. Therefore, it seemed appropriate to study contrast induced coronary hyperemia after intracoronary administration of verapamil.

In the present study, the nonionic iohexol-140 was compared with the extensively studied ionic contrast agent diatrizoate (Urographin^R). Because the most important characteristic of a contrast agent for imaging purposes is its iodine content, for fair comparison a similarly low iodinated, but still hypertonic 30% dilution of this last agent was selected (table A.1).

A.2 Methods

A.2.1 Animal preparation and instrumentation

After premedication with 1 cc Thalamonal^R (0.05 mg fentanyl and 2.5 mg droperidol) eight dogs of either sex (average weight 31 kg, range 22-48 kg) were anesthetized with intravenous pentobarbital (25 mg/kg) and ventilated with room air by an Ångstrom respirator. A left thoracotomy was performed through the fifth intercostal space and right or left atrial epicardial pacing electrodes were sutured in place. The proximal left anterior descending coronary artery was dissected free and encircled with an electromagnetic flow probe (Skalar Transflow 601) and a snare occluder distal of the flow probe to establish zero flow and to assess reactive hyperemia as a test for the integrity of the preparation. After dissection of both femoral arteries, a pigtail tipmanometer catheter (Millar Microtip catheter pressure transducer PC 474 A) was advanced into the left ventricle. After administration of 5000 U heparin intravenously, a 5F left Judkins catheter was used to selectively cannulate the left main coronary artery under fluoroscopic guidance. The position of the coronary catheter was not varied during the study.

A.2.2   Contrast injections

After determination of reactive hyperemia following a 20 seconds occlusion, injections of 2, 4 and 6 ml iohexol and 6 ml diatrizoate were administered into the left coronary artery of each dog. Each dosage was administered three times; the sequence of injections was randomized. All contrast injections were performed at a constant injection speed of 4 ml/s using an angiographic contrast injector (Sybron Angiomat 300). To ensure exact knowledge of the onset of injection, an electrical pulse signal corresponding with the movement of the injector barrel was recorded. Each injection was performed only on the premises that the basic hemodynamic parameters had returned to control conditions as at the beginning of the experiment and at least a 2 minutes pause after the former injection was regarded. Each sequence was concluded by another 20 seconds occlusion of the coronary artery.

To test the calcium ion entry hypothesis, the whole sequence was repeated 30 minutes after intracoronary administration of 0.5 mg verapamil when coronary flow had returned to control values in all dogs.

A.2.3   Hemodynamic recordings

ECG, left ventricular pressure, left ventricular peak positive dP/dt ($(dP/dt)_{max}$), phasic and mean coronary blood flow, and the injector pulse were recorded, using an 8 channels recorder (Hewlett Packard). Animal body temperature, carbon dioxide content of end-expiratory air (Gould Godart Capnograph Mark II), and the fluid balance of the dog were carefully monitored to prevent changes in hemodynamic parameters as a result of shifts in body temperature, pH, or state of hydration. During the 20 seconds occlusion period, at the conclusion of each sequence of injections, electrical zero was matched to occlusive zero.

Table A.2: *Baseline values (mean ± S.D.).*

	before verapamil	after verapamil
coronary blood flow (ml/min)	47 ± 33	47 ± 28
left ventricular $(dP/dt)_{max}$ (mmHg/s)	2662 ± 705	2188 ± 628
systolic left ventricular pressure (mmHg)	131 ± 25	117 ± 11
heart rate (beats/min)	169 ± 13	167 ± 14

A.2.4 Statistical analysis

To determine the statistical significance of the changes in hemodynamic parameters compared to control values, and for comparison of these parameters before and after intracoronary administration of verapamil, the Student t-test for paired observations was used. To assess the reaction to the three injections of the same dose of a contrast agent in the same dog under similar conditions, coefficients of variation were calculated. For the relation between changes in mean coronary blood blow and change in $(dP/dt)_{max}$ after contrast injection, individual correlation coefficients were calculated for each dog, using the least square regression method. All values are presented as mean ± 1 standard deviation and a p-value of less than 0.05 was considered significant.

A.3 Results

A.3.1 Baseline values and reactions to verapamil

Baseline values are presented in table A.2. During the experiment these values were not affected by the presence of the tip of the Judkins catheter in the ostium of the left coronary artery.

After intracoronary administration of 0.5 mg verapamil as a bolus injection, an increase in coronary blood flow was observed to $302 \pm 72\%$ of the control value with its maximum after 58 ± 19 seconds. In all dogs this was accompanied by a significant decrease in left ventricular systolic pressure and left ventricular $(dP/dt)_{max}$ ($p < 0.01$). The influence on heart rate was variable and ranged from -16 to $+12$ beats per minute. Coronary blood flow returned to control values within 20 minutes af-

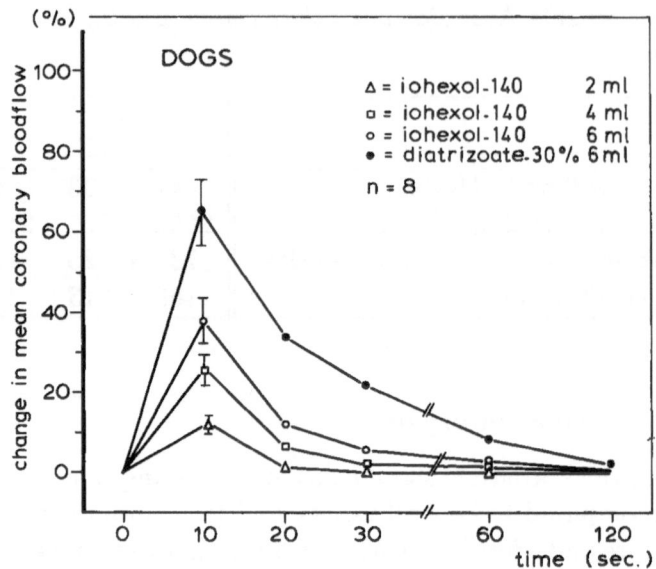

Figure A.1: *Changes in mean coronary blood flow during the first two minutes after contrast injection.*

ter verapamil administration. Left ventricular systolic pressure and left ventricular $(dP/dt)_{max}$, however, remained depressed (table A.2).

A.3.2   Effect of contrast injections on coronary blood flow

In response to the contrast injections, a reproducible reaction of coronary blood flow could be seen, consisting of an early dip followed by a subsequent increase. Qualitatively, this pattern was not different from observations by other investigators [4, 8, 9]. The early dip was seen within 5 seconds and the maximal hyperemic effect was observed about 10 seconds after the start of the contrast injection (figure A.1). The effect of diatrizoate is not only more vigorous but also lasts longer ($p < 0.01$).

The effect of iohexol on coronary flow appears to be dose related and is significant for all doses (figure A.2); the effect is small compared with all former investigations to the effect of contrast injections on coronary blood flow: $12.3 \pm 7.1\%, 25.6 \pm 11.1\%$ and $38.2 \pm 16.7\%$ after 2 ml, 4 ml and 6 ml iohexol, respectively ($p < 0.01$ for all doses). After diluted diatrizoate, the maximal increase in mean coronary blood flow averaged $65.2 \pm 23.7\%$, significantly exceeding the values as observed after iohexol

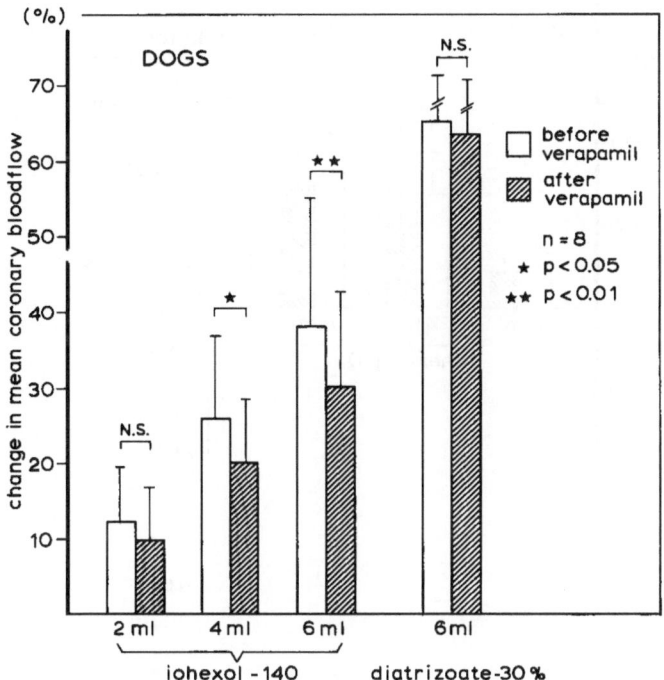

Figure A.2: *Influence of contrast injections on mean coronary blood flow before and after intracoronary administration of 0.5 mg verapamil (N.S. = not significant).*

($p < 0.01$).

Following the intracoronary administration of verapamil, the hyperemic response to iohexol decreased to $9.8 \pm 2.0\%$ (not significant), $20.0 \pm 3.0\%$ ($p < 0.05$) and $29.9 \pm 12.8\%$ ($p < 0.01$), respectively (figure A.2). The reaction to diatrizoate, however, was not affected by verapamil ($63.3 \pm 39.3\%$).

A.3.3 Effect of contrast injections on left ventricular $(dP/dt)_{max}$, left ventricular systolic pressure, and heart rate

Changes in $(dP/dt)_{max}$ were studied as representative for changes in the inotropic state of the myocardium. After intracoronary injection of all

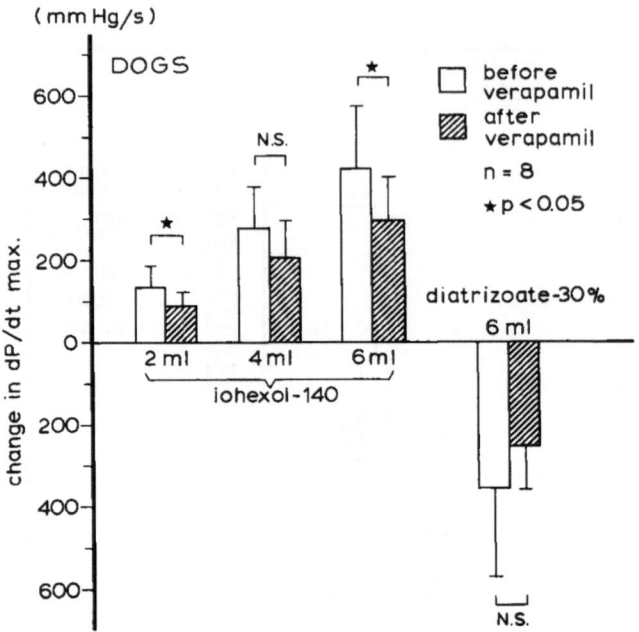

Figure A.3: *Influence of contrast injections on left ventricular* $(dP/dt)_{max}$ *before and after intracoronary administration of 0.5 mg verapamil.*

doses of iohexol, a significant increase in $(dP/dt)_{max}$ was observed: 131 ± 52 mm Hg/s, 275 ± 102 mm Hg/s, and 417 ± 156 mm Hg/s, respectively ($p < 0.01$ for all doses) while a significant decrease of 363 ± 210 mm Hg/s was observed after injection of 6 ml diatrizoate ($p < 0.01$). This initial decrease of $(dP/dt)_{max}$ after diatrizoate injection was followed by a slight increase a few seconds later as described before [5]. After intracoronary administration of verapamil, the change in $(dP/dt)_{max}$ decreased to 89 ± 29 mm Hg/s ($p < 0.05$), 205 ± 83 mm Hg/s (N.S.) and 295 ± 105 mm Hg/s ($p < 0.05$) after injection of 2 ml, 4 ml, and 6 ml iohexol, respectively (figure A.3). The reaction of $(dP/dt)_{max}$ to diatrizoate, however, was not significantly altered by verapamil (-255 ± 109 mm Hg/s, N.S.).

The effects on left ventricular systolic pressure parallelled those on $(dP/dt)_{max}$ although the influence of verapamil was not significant (figure A.4). Heart rate remained unchanged after intracoronary injection of either dose of iohexol. After diatrizoate, however, in most dogs a

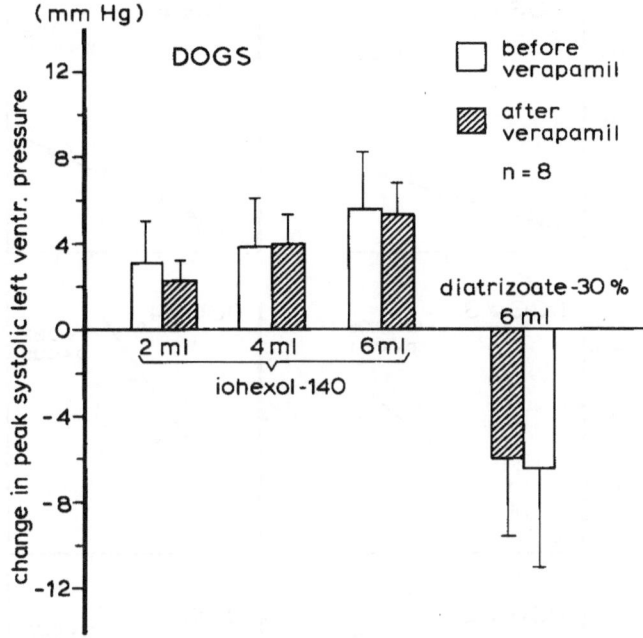

Figure A.4: *Influence of contrast injections on peak systolic left ventricular pressure before and after intracoronary administration of 0.5 mg verapamil.*

slight acceleration was seen necessitating overpacing to ensure a constant heart rate.

A.3.4 Reaction to 20 seconds coronary artery occlusion

Coronary flow reserve determined by a 20 seconds occlusion period was similar for all dogs at the beginning and at the end of every sequence of contrast injections (table A.3). After administration of verapamil, however, coronary blood flow reserve decreased from $356 \pm 59\%$ to $285 \pm 55\%$ ($p < 0.05$). During occlusion, predictable changes were seen in left ventricular peak positive and peak negative dP/dt, indicating an impairment of myocardial contractile state and a decrease of left ventricular pressure as described before [4, 5].

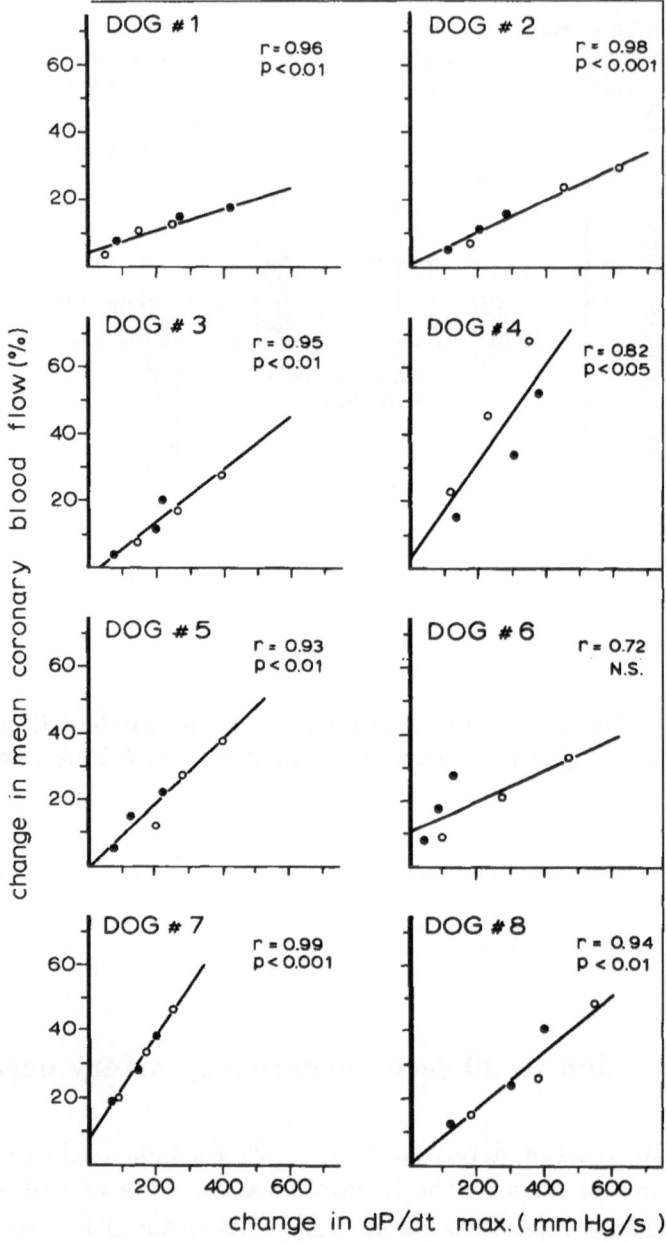

Figure A.5: *Correlations between changes in mean coronary blood flow after contrast injection and changes in left ventricular* $(dP/dt)_{max}$ *for each dog. Open and closed circles represent values before and after verapamil administration, respectively. Each point represents the mean value of three corresponding determinations.*

Table A.3: *Maximal hyperemic flow after 20 seconds of occlusion, expressed as the percentage of the baseline value (mean ± S.D.).*

	before verapamil	after verapamil
before series of 12 contrast injections	356 ± 59	285 ± 55
after series of 12 contrast injections	345 ± 50	289 ± 61

A.3.5 Relation between change in coronary blood flow and change in left ventricular $(dP/dt)_{max}$

Considering the fact that the isotonic contrast agent iohexol 140 did not influence heart rate and taking into account the observation that the contrast induced increase in coronary blood flow was diminished after verapamil administration, the relation between change in mean coronary blood flow and left ventricular $(dP/dt)_{max}$ was further investigated. For this purpose, the observed changes of coronary blood flow after the different doses of iohexol before and after verapamil were plotted against the corresponding change in $(dP/dt)_{max}$ (figure A.5). For each dog correlation coefficients were computed. Because the reactions to the three similar iohexol injections in the same sequence were invariably close together in each dog, as indicated by small coefficients of variation (mean $\pm$ SD $= 0.05 \pm 0.03$), only the mean values of three similar determinations are plotted in figure A.5.

Because the range of the baseline values for coronary blood flow is rather large due to the differences in animal body weight and size of the left anterior descending artery, while the baseline values for $(dP/dt)_{max}$ are in the same range (table A.2), the change in coronary flow is presented as a percentage in figure A.5, while the change in $(dP/dt)_{max}$ is presented as an absolute value. For all but one dogs there is a significant positive correlation between increase in coronary blood flow and increase in inotropic state as represented by $(dP/dt)_{max}$ ($r = 0.91 \pm 0.09$).

A.4 Discussion

In addition to the information about the pathoanatomy, the coronary arteriogram provides valuable pathophysiologic data. The time parameters of the transport of contrast medium constitute an indicator of myocardial perfusion. Calculation of these time parameters from myocardial time-density curves to quantitate coronary blood flow, however, is only meaningful if flow remains constant throughout the acquisition period of the curve.

The currently used contrast agents induce considerable hyperemia within seconds after injection thus interfering with a correct interpretation of the time-density curve and calculation of the mean transit time. For this reason, a number of investigators used other time parameters such as appearance time, and represented the vascular volume by maximal contrast intensity [10, 11, 12, 13, 14]. It would be more elegant, however, to use a contrast agent without noticeable influence on flow and this was the reason why the present experiment were performed.

Intracoronary injection of a hypertonic, not easily diffusible solution causes morphologic changes, transient sludging, and aggregation of red blood cells resulting in an initial fall in flow followed by an increase 5-20 seconds after injection [8, 15]. In case of classical ionic contrast agents, this is accompanied by a marked transient depression in left ventricular $(dP/dt)_{max}$ and left ventricular pressure. The newer nonionic and generally less hypertonic agents, on the other hand, produce a slight initial increase in $(dP/dt)_{max}$, being indirectly responsible for an accessory increase in coronary blood flow. The reason for these changes in inotropic state are not yet completely understood. Intracoronary contrast injection leads to complex electrolyte shifts due to dilution of the plasma ions by the contrast medium itselve, to water shift caused by hyperosmolality, and due to sodium content and calcium chelation in case of ionic agents [5]. Consequently, myocardial depression after intracoronary administration of ionic agents is explained by an imbalance between Na^+ and Ca^{++} in myocardial extracellular fluid, competing for membrane transport into the muscle cell and for participation in regulation of myocardial contractile state [15]. This is accompanied by an increase in the Na^+/Ca^{++} ratio in coronary sinus blood which is temporally related to the myocardial depression [5, 16]. On the other hand, the positive inotropic effect of the nonionic agents is at least partly attributed to a temporary increase in Ca^{++} concentration and improved excitation - contraction coupling in the heart muscle and is accompanied by a decreased Na^+/Ca^{++} ratio in coronary sinus blood [5]. None of the explanations, however, is completely satisfactory and many questions remain unsolved.

If the rise in $(dP/dt)_{max}$ and an associated secondary rise in coronary blood flow is mediated by Ca^{++} ions, this increase should be partially blocked by Ca^{++} entry blocking drugs. Of all calcium blockers, verapamil has the best established effect on the myocytes and lacks direct effects on peripheral vascular resistance and afterload when administered intracoronary [17]; for this reason, this drug was chosen to verify the hypothesis that the hyperemic response to iohexol can be diminished in this way.

In the present experiment a moderate but significant decrease in hyperemic response to iohexol injection after intracoronary administration of 0.5 mg verapamil could be confirmed. Verapamil did not influence the response to diatrizoate, suggesting a different mechanism for the negative inotropic action of ionic agents. Moreover, the equality of the response to diatrizoate before and after verapamil argues against unforeseen changes in our preparation.

Because the nonionic contrast agent used - iohexol 140 - is not hyperosmolal and does not influence heart rate, it seems attractive to explain the induced hyperemia directly by its positive inotropic effect. For this reason, the relationship between both parameters was examined and was linear and significant in all but one dogs. Furthermore, in all dogs the regression line almost passes through the origin, suggesting that no other important factor is responsible for the hyperemic response to iohexol.

Although these investigations provide some answers to the problems stated, new questions arise as well. Considering the explanation for the early dip in blood flow immediately after the injection of hyperosmolal solutions as stated above [8], we cannot explain that this dip also occurred after injection of an iso-osmolal solution.

Other questions concern the maximally acceptable hyperemia and the minimally required amount of injected contrast agent to provide an image quality sufficient to obtain acceptable images. For the time being, 6-8 ml of a low iodinated agent, injected at a speed of 4 ml/s, is the minimum.

Finally, the diminished coronary flow reserve after verapamil needs an explanation. Following the release of a 20 seconds coronary occlusion the coronary bed is maximally dilated and consequently peak flow is pressure dependent [18]. After verapamil, aortic pressure is about 10% lower, which means that the lower coronary perfusion pressure is at least partly responsible for the decrease in coronary flow reserve.

A.5   Conclusion

From this study it can be concluded that intracoronary injection of iohexol 140 induces an increase in coronary blood flow, which is dose
related and only moderate in comparison with all other present contrast
agents. This reaction is partly correlated to an increase in myocardial
inotropic state and can be significantly diminished by previous intracoronary administration of verapamil. This means that the isotonic nonionic
contrast medium iohexol 140 (Omnipaque 140^R) brings closer a reliable
assessment of time parameters from myocardial time-density curves and
is a further step in the identification of the contrast agent of choice for
quantitative myocardial videodensitometry.

References

[1] Ziedzes des Plantes B G. Eine roentgenographische Methode zur separaten
    Abbildung bestimmter Teile des Objekts. *Fortschr Roentgenstr*, 52:69–79,
    1935.

[2] Van der Werf T, Heethaar R M, Stegehuis H, and Meijler F L. The concept
    of apparent cardiac arrest as a prerequisite for coronary digital subtraction
    angiography. *J Am Coll Cardiol*, 4:239–244, 1984.

[3] Zierler K L. *Circulation times and the theory of indicator dilution methods
    for determining blood flow and volume*, pages 585–615. American Physio-
    logical Society, Washington DC, 1962.

[4] Gerber K H and Higgins C B. Comparative effects of ionic and nonionic
    contrast materials on coronary and peripheral blood flow. *Invest Radiol*,
    17:292–298, 1982.

[5] Schræder R, Baller D, Hoeft A, Korb H, Wolpers H G, and Hellige G.
    Reduced side effects of low osmolality nonionic contrast media in coro-
    nary arteriography. In V Taenzer and E Zeitler, editors, *Contrast me-
    dia in urography, angiography and computerized tomography*, pages 67–77.
    George Thieme Verlag, Stutgart, New York, 1983.

[6] Simon R, Koch M, Hermann G, Amende I, and Lichtlen P R. Direct effects
    of an ionic nonionic contrast agent on the coronary circulation in man. In
    Proceedings Xth World Congress Cardiology, page 294. Washington, 1986.

[7] Wilson R F, Laughlin D E, Ackell P H, Chilian W M, Holida M D, Hart-
    ley C J, Armstrong M L, Marcus M L, and White C W. Transluminal
    subselective measurement of coronary artery blood flow velocity and va-
    sodilator reserve in man. *Circulation*, 72:82–92, 1985.

[8] Hodgson J M B, Mancini G B J, Legrand V, and Vogel R A. Characterization of changes in coronary blood flow during the first six seconds after intracoronary contrast injection. *Invest Radiol*, 20:246–252, 1985.

[9] Friedman H Z, De Boe S F, Mc Gillem M J, and Mancini G B J. The immediate effects of iohexol on coronary blood flow and myocardial function in vivo. *Circulation*, 74:1416–1423, 1986.

[10] Vogel R, LeFree M, Bates E, O'Neill W, Foster R, Kirlin P, Smith D, and Pitt B. Application of digital techniques to selective coronary arteriography: use of myocardial appearance time to measure coronary flow reserve. *Am Heart J*, 107:153–164, 1984.

[11] O'Neill W W, Walton J A, Bates E R, Colfer H T, Aueron F M, LeFree M T, Pitt B, and Vogel R A. Criteria for successful coronary angioplasty as assessed by alterations in coronary vasodilatory reserve. *J Am Coll Cardiol*, 3:1382–1390, 1984.

[12] Nissen S E, Elion J L, Booth D C, Evans J, and DeMaria A N. Value and limitations of computer analysis of digital subtraction angiography in the assessment of coronary flow reserve. *Circulation*, 73:562–571, 1986.

[13] Hodgson J M, Legrand V, Bates E R, Mancini G B J, Aueron F M, O'Neill W W, Simon S B, Beauman G J, LeFree M T, and Vogel R A. Validation in dogs of a rapid digital angiographic technique to measure relative coronary blood flow during routine cardiac catheterization. *Am J Cardiol*, 55:188–193, 1985.

[14] Vogel R A. *Functional Imaging of the Coronary Circulation Using Digital Radiography*, pages 175–188. 1986.

[15] Gerber K H, Higgins C B, Yuh Y, and Koziol J A. Regional myocardial hemodynamic and metabolic effects of ionic and nonionic contrast media in normal and ischemic states. *Circulation*, 65:1307–1314, 1982.

[16] Higgins C B and Schmidt W. Alterations in calcium levels of coronary sinus blood during coronary arteriography in the dog. *Circulation*, 58:512–519, 1978.

[17] Walsh R A, Badke F R, and O'Rourke R A. Differential effects of systemic and intracoronary calcium channel blocking agents on global and regional left ventricular function in conscious dogs. *Am Heart J*, 102:341–350, 1981.

[18] Hoffman J I E. Maximal coronary flow and the concept of coronary vascular reserve. *Circulation*, 70:153–159, 1984.

Appendix B

Fitting Procedures for Time-Density Curves

The sampled average pixel densities in a region of interest in a series of images (called a *study*) are corrected by subtraction of the average densities in a corresponding background region of interest of identical shape and size. The remaining curve constitutes a sampled dilution curve superposed upon a baseline density a_0 and starts to be different from zero at time t_0 (figure B.1).

The sampled data are fitted by an appropriate mathematical function, $y(t)$, defined as follows:

$$
\begin{aligned}
y(t) &= a_0 + f(t) & t \geq t_0 \\
y(t) &= a_0 & t < t_0
\end{aligned}
\tag{B.1}
$$

The function $f(t)$, defined for $t \geq t_0$, is the gamma function $g(t)$ or the lognormal function $h(t)$:

$$
g(t) = D_{max} \cdot \Theta^a \cdot e^{-a(\Theta - 1)}
\tag{B.2}
$$

$$
h(t) = D_{max} \cdot e^{-b \ln^2 \Theta},
\tag{B.3}
$$

with

$$
\begin{aligned}
D_{max} &= \text{maximal value for contrast density of the sampled data} \\
\Theta &= (t - t_0)/(t_{max} - t_0) \\
t_{max} &= \text{time of maximal contrast density} \\
a \text{ and } b &\quad \text{are shaping factors}
\end{aligned}
$$

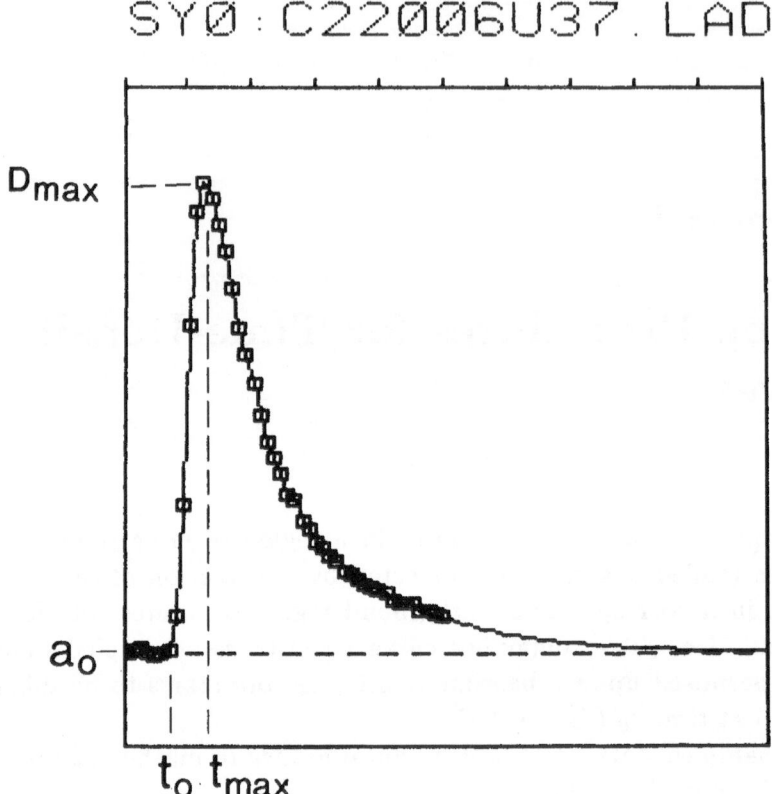

Figure B.1: *Background corrected time-density curve (squares), the best gam-mafit (drawn line) and the parameters necessary to obtain this fit. a_0 = baseline density level, t_0 = time at which the ascending part of the curve starts, D_{max} = maximal contrast intensity, t_{max} = time corresponding with D_{max}.*

The function $y(t)$ in equation (B.1) is determined by the five param-eters a_0, t_0, D_{max} and t_{max} and a or b respectively, and fits the sampled data according to the Marquardt method [1, 2]. All samples between $t = 0$ and the moment at which the descending part of the curve becomes less than 60% of D_{max}, are used for curve fitting. The parameters a_0, D_{max}, t_{max}, Θ and a or b are determined in an iterative way such that the relative error between the observed data and the fit are minimized. The quality of the fit is judged by this relative error E_r which is defined

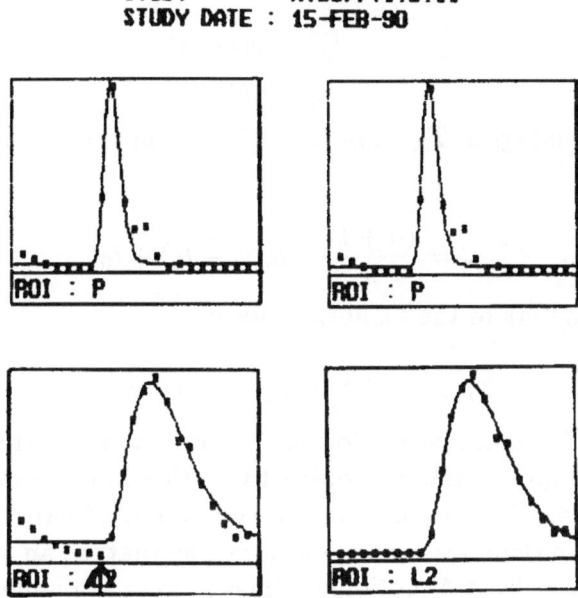

Figure B.2: *Example of manual instead of automatic indication of the baseline level a_0.*

as:

$$E_r = \left\{ \frac{\sum_{i=1}^{k} [y(t_i) - y_i]^2}{\sum_{i=1}^{k} [y(t_i) - a_0]^2} \right\}^{1/2} \times 100\% \qquad (B.4)$$

where y_i is the sampled density in the i^{st} image and k is the total number of images in the study. In all studies, a 10% value of E_r was considered as the upper limit for acceptance of the fit as being representative for the sampled data.

Evaluation of the accuracy of the fits was performed by comparison of the relative errors and by determination of T_{mn} in 9 consecutive studies in 3 afferent ROIs and in 4 capillary ROIs at a fixed flow rate of 200 ml/min in the flow model described in chapter 5. The relative error was slightly smaller for the lognormal fit, the gamma fit produced a better reproducibility [3].

Mean transit time was calculated from the fit according to theory by equation:

$$T_{mn} = \frac{\int_0^\infty t \cdot y(t) \cdot dt}{\int_0^\infty \cdot y(t) \cdot dt} \tag{B.5}$$

By solving this integral, T_{mn} can be expressed in the parameters of the gammafit as:

$$T_{mn} = \frac{(a+1)}{a} \cdot (t_{max} - t_0) + t_0 \tag{B.6}$$

or in the parameters of the lognormal fit as:

$$T_{mn} = e^{3/4b} \cdot (t_{max} - t_0) + t_0 \tag{B.7}$$

One kind of manual correction for the fit was permitted in the human studies (chapter 7 and 8): contrast injection in these studies always started 7 seconds after the inspiration command. Mostly a deep inspiration lasted less than 3 seconds, which means that, at an average heart rate of 80/min, at least 5 motionless images were available before start of contrast injection to provide a stable baseline level. Sometimes, however, inspiration lasted longer and in a few of these cases problems were encountered in determination of the baseline density (zero level). If the baseline was clearly discernible by the remaining sample points, manual correction of the baseline was permitted by indicating the parameter a_0. An example of such a correction is presented in figure B.2. If any doubt remained, the curves were rejected.

References

[1] Bevington P R. *Data reduction and error analysis for the physical sciences,* pages 204–246. McGraw-Hill, New York, 1969.

[2] Press W H, Flannery B P, Tenkolsky S A, and Vettering W T. *Numerical recipes. The art of scientific computing,* pages 523–528. Cambridge University Press, Cambridge, 1987.

[3] Uijen G H J, Pijls N H J, and Van der Werf T. The accuracy of densitometric time parameters in the analysis of myocardial perfusion. In *Computers in Cardiology 1988,* pages 215–218. IEEE Computer Society, Washington DC, 1989.

Summary

In this book a new approach is described to assess myocardial perfusion by videodensitometry. In contrary to all former approaches in this field, efforts to calculate resting blood flow or coronary flow reserve (CFR) have been abandoned. Instead, maximally achievable flow through the myocardium is considered as the most relevant parameter representing the clinical status of the patient and it is this parameter which we tried to assess in our studies.

After injection of contrast agent into a coronary artery, temporal changes in myocardial contrast density can be studied as a function of time, resulting in a so-called time-density curve (TDC). This curve resembles an indicator dilution curve and contains information about myocardial blood flow. Previous attemps to derive information about flow from these TDCs, have been hampered by a number of serious problems, necessitating the assumption of unproven - and untrue - hypotheses and violation of physiological principles. In this book, these problems could be either solved or circumvented. Accurate calculation of mean transit time (T_{mn}) of contrast passage at maximal hyperemia proved to be possible, whereafter maximal flow could be predicted in a reliable and reproducible way.

In contrary to clinical methods to calculate CFR, always crude, laborious and mostly violating fundamental principles of physiology, an accurate method is provided for assessment of maximal perfusion through arbitrary parts of the myocardium. This method is strictly in accordance with the original principles of indicator dilution theory.

In **chapter 1** the fundamental shortcomings of classical coronary arteriography to evaluate the functional significance of a stenosis in a coronary artery are explained and the need for a functional instead of an anatomical interpretation of the coronary arteriogram is emphasized.

The best way to assess the real significance of a stenosis is to study its effect on blood flow. In contrary to the results in the animal laboratory, however, use of CFR in clinical practice has been disappointing because of the many confounding factors influencing resting flow and CFR, but not related to the stenosis itself.

Because most patients with angina pectoris are not complaining about insufficient resting flow or CFR, but about inadequate maximal flow, achievable by (a part of) their myocardium, maximal flow is proposed as the most relevant parameter to reflect the functional status of a patient from a clinical point of view.

In **chapter 2**, an overview is presented of a number of methods used to calculate coronary flow or myocardial perfusion in the animal laboratory (timed venous collection, electromagnetic flow measurement, epicardial ultrasonic flow velocity measurement, microspheres) and in clinical practice (coronary sinus thermodilution, gas clearance methods, the Doppler catheter, videodensitometry, positron emission tomography). Mechanisms, backgrounds, advantages, and limitations of these methods are shortly described.

In **chapter 3** the applications of indicator dilution theory in the investigation of the cardiovascular system are summarized. Because of the paramount importance of knowledge of the background theory to understand and appreciate the remaining part of this book, the relations between flow, vascular volume, and mean transit time are derived and explained. Videodensitometry or digital arteriography is defined as studying passage of contrast agent through the myocardium as a function of time by analysis of temporal changes in density. This is considered as an application of indicator dilution theory to the coronary circulation. Study of contrast passage has become possible by applying principles of digital subtraction during ECG- triggered image acquisition.

In **chapter 4** the many problems, encountered in videodensitometry, are discussed. The most serious problems concern 1. the influence of the contrast agent (the indicator) on flow (the parameter to be measured), resulting in flow changes during the acquisition of the TDC; 2. changes in vascular volume between different situations in which flow is compared; 3. difficulties in the determination of T_{mn} due to insufficient image quality, and 4. measurement of contrast density instead of contrast concentration.

Previous methods to assess flow by videodensitometry and their inherent shortcomings are briefly described, such as substitution of T_{mn} by other time parameters and representation of vascular volume by maximal contrast intensity. Two major suggestions are put forward to solve these problems. In the first place, all studies should be performed at maximal coronary and myocardial hyperemia, thus excluding changes in flow and volume and assuring a linear relation between density and concentration of the contrast agent. In the second place, image quality should be improved in such a way that T_{mn} can be calculated unequivocally from the TDC. This can be achieved by extensive training to hold breath prior to the catheterization to avoid motion artifacts, and by a special way of ECG-triggering, called apparent cardiac arrest, which means that X-ray pulses are in synchrony with the triggered heart rate.

In **chapter 5** a number of theoretical considerations from the former chapters are tested in a hydrodynamic flow model, in which flow and volume can be controlled and in which perfect digital subtraction is possible because of the absence of motion. The empirical value of different time parameters, used to calculate flow ratios between different situations, is tested. As predicted by theory, T_{mn} proved to be the best parameter for this purpose. Appearance time (T_{app}) was not reliable, especially not at lower flow rates. Using T_{mn}, absolute flow could be predicted in this model as well, because the volume was exactly known.

In this flow model, also some physical and mathematical problems could be studied. Applicability of Lambert-Beer's law to the practical situation in the catheterization laboratory could be verified, which means that a linear relation was established between the amount of iodine in a perpendicular section and the density value assigned to this section. Curve fitting procedures, using the lognormal and the gamma function, could also be tested.

In **chapter 6** the suitability of inverse mean transit time to predict flow, was validated in an animal study. In 8 dogs, a ring-mounted epicardial Doppler probe was implanted around the left circumflex artery (LCx) and a balloon occluder was placed just distal to the Doppler probe for induction of different degrees of stenosis. Pacing electrodes to provide ECG- triggered image acquisition were fixed on the left atrial appendage. The dogs were catheterized in the catheterization laboratory 7-10 days later and ECG-triggered digital subtraction studies of contrast passage were performed at different degrees of LCx stenosis. During these studies, maximal coronary and myocardial hyperemia was induced by continuous infusion of dipyridamole. From the contrast passage curves (time density curves) obtained from the myocardium supplied by the LCx artery, T_{mn} was calculated and correlated to flow velocity as measured by the Doppler probe. The Dopper probes were calibrated against an EM flow probe shortly before sacrifice. An excellent relation proved to be present between relative maximal flow calculated by videodensitometry and real flow over the complete range from 0 to 174 ± 42 ml/min ($r = 0.97$).

Because flow in this animal model was not influenced by the contrast agent, and because the vascular volume remained constant during the whole experiment, this model offered an ideal possibility to test in vivo the validity of the former hypotheses concerning substitution of T_{mn} by T_{app} and maximal contrast density (D_{max}) as an index of volume. Only a poor correlation between $1/T_{app}$ and flow was found, while D_{max} did not remain constant but rather decreased with decreasing flow. Using the D_{max}/T_{app} ratio, better results were obtained than in using both parameters separately. These results, however, were still inferior to the results obtained by the physiological time parameter T_{mn}.

From this animal validation study it can be concluded that accurate calculation of relative maximal myocardial perfusion by videodensitometry is feasible in the intact living being, using mean transit time and strictly in accordance with the principles of indicator dilution theory.

In **chapter 7** we tried to apply the achievements of the animal study in conscious man. The ideal model to study changes in flow as a result of changes in the severity of a coronary artery stenosis, is provided by percutaneous transluminal coronary angioplasty (PTCA). In order to correlate improvement in perfusion to functional instead of anatomic parameters we selected 40 consecutive patients with angina pectoris, a clearly positive exercise stress test (ET), and single vessel disease at coronary arteriography less than 6 weeks before the intervention. Exercise testing was repeated shortly before the PTCA and 7-10 days thereafter. The patients were extensively instructed to hold breath and to remain motionless during image acquisition to ensure an image quality well enough to determine T_{mn} reliably. Maximal hyperemia was induced by intracoronary administration of papaverine 30 seconds before start of image acquisition. T_{mn} at maximal hyperemia was calculated before and after PTCA for the dilated vessel as well as for the remaining, apparently normal, vessels. The relative increase in myocardial flow, obtained by the PTCA, was represented by the ratio of T_{mn} before and after PTCA, according to the results of the animal study. This ratio was called the maximal flow ratio (MFR). Unlike coronary flow reserve, this maximal flow ratio is not dependent on heart rate, previous infarction in other segments, left ventricular hypertrophy, the PTCA procedure itself, or other confounding variables. It is only dependent on arterial pressure which can easily be measured and corrected for as was done in this study.

In this particular study population, the predictive value of exercise testing was almost 100%. Therefore exercise testing could be used as the gold standard of functional success or failure of the PTCA. MFR of more or less than 1.6 was related to presence or absence of reversal of ET result from positive to negative. The value of 1.6 was determined by discriminant analysis. By calculation of MFR, immediately after the PTCA, a correct classification of the result as successful or unsuccessful according to ET results, was present in 94% of all cases. When using anatomic criteria (decrease of area stenosis of $\geq$ 20% and residual stenosis < 50%) or final transstenotic pressure gradient ($\leq$ 15 mm Hg) as predictor of successful PTCA, a correct classification could be made only in 66% and 74% of all cases respectively.

Because all patients in this study had 2 normal vessels, values of T_{mn} at maximal hyperemia for these vessels could be obtained as well. It turned out that a definite range exists of what can be called a normal T_{mn} at maximal hyperemia. Moreover, values of T_{mn}, corresponding with successfully dilated vessels, returned completely to normal.

From this study in patients, it can be concluded that improvement in maximal myocardial flow as reflected by decrease of T_{mn} at maximal hyperemia, shows an excellent correlation with the functional result of the PTCA. Because this calculation can be performed on-line, with the patient still on the table and the catheter still in situ, it can be used for decision making during the course of the procedure.

In **chapter 8** the reproducibility of T_{mn} determination in man is further evaluated. In 20 patients, two identical studies of either the LCA or the RCA were performed with an interval of 5- 10 minutes and the reproducibility of the total chain from image acquisition to image processing, curve processing, and the final calculation of T_{mn}, was tested. Reproducibility proved to be excellent with a correlation coefficient of 0.98 between the first and second measurement.

In **chapter 9** a general discussion is presented and the following **conclusions** are drawn:

A. Assessment of maximal myocardial blood flow can be performed accurately by videodensitometry, using mean transit time as a parameter of flow. This can be done strictly in accordance with the principles of the indicator dilution theory.

B. In this way, a reliable method is provided to evaluate changes in maximal flow, as a result of an intervention. This evaluation can be performed on-line. In case of a PTCA, it can be used therefore for decision making during the course of the procedure. Increase in maximal flow, achievable by the myocardium supplied by the dilated artery, is the best correlate of functional improvement of the patient.

C. Ranges of normal values of mean transit time at maximal hyperemia can be discriminated. Therefore, this method can be used during routine diagnostic cardiac catheterization to obtain information about the functional significance of a stenosis in a coronary artery by one single contrast injection at maximal hyperemia.

D. After successful PTCA, minimal resistance to flow through the dilated lesion immediately returns to normal.

In **appendix A** a study about the hemodynamic effects of contrast injection is presented. It is a pilot study performed before the other studies and searched for a contrast agent without effect on myocardial blood flow. For this reason the isotonic isoviscous contrast agent iohexol-140 was tested. Although the hemodynamic effects caused by this agent were much less than those of any other contrast agent, an increase in flow of approximately 40% was still observed when using the minimally acceptable dosage for sufficient image quality in the anesthetized dog. In humans, even a higher concentration has to be used. Although it is still true that the contrast agent with least influence on flow is the most preferable one, this approach was left after the decision to restrict ourselves to study maximal flow only. Under this condition the hyperemic response to contrast agent is of no concern anymore.

In **appendix B**, at last, the curve fitting procedures by a lognormal and a gamma function as used in these studies, are described.

Index

^{133}Xe, 19
^{13}N-ammonia, 21
^{82}Rb, 21
^{82}Rb generator, 22

absorption characteristics, 57
accuracy, 169
acquisition rate, 65
acquisition time, 55, 65
Al filter, 56
angina pectoris, 5
angiographic success, 112
apparent cardiac arrest, 47, 75
appearance time (T_{app}), xvi, 27, 46, 57, 59,
    65, 66, 72, 92, 93, 119, 142, 162
  different definitions, 78
Ar, 19
area stenosis, 112
  reduction of, 108
  residual, 108, 112
arteriolar vessels, 4
aspirin, 103
atherosclerosis
  progression, 147
  regression, 147
atrial fibrillation, 109
atrial pacing, 45, 109, 153
atropine, 73
attenuation of radiation, 44
automatic brightness control, 75, 104

background, 47, 55, 57
background corrected curve, 82

background correction, 47, 82
background density, 47, 56, 57, 78, 86, 91
balloon occluder, 73, 75
baseline density, 104, 167, 168, 170
blood temperature, 19
breath-holding, 45–47, 102, 117, 130, 138
build up time (T_{bu}), 46, 58, 59
bypass grafts, 14, 121, 146
bypass surgery, 95, 146

Ca^{++} dependency, 153, 154
Ca^{++} entry blocking drugs, 163
calibration, 14–17, 55, 57, 58, 82
capillary entrapment, 16
carbon dioxide, 154
cardiac catheterization
  diagnostic, 143
chemotoxic effect, 152
chi-square test, 108
cineangiography, 2
collateral circulation, 2, 5, 102, 121, 144,
  146
concentration-time curve, 29
contractile function, 144, 147
contrast agent, 32, 33, 40, 42, 43, 63, 75,
  94, 101, 141
  nonionic, 104
contrast concentration, 43, 44, 142
contrast density, xv, 21, 33, 43, 44, 46,
  119, 142, 167
  maximal (D_{max}), xv, 72, 81, 89, 92, 94,
  142, 162, 168

time of maximal (T_{max}), 59, 66, 78, 167, 168
contrast echocardiography, 22
contrast injection, 4, 46, 55, 75, 92, 104, 118, 130, 156, 157
  subselective, 142
contrast passage, 8, 19, 33, 39, 40, 45, 46, 71, 72, 141
control vessels, 116, 117, 120
coronary arteries
  normal, 120, 142
coronary arteriography, 1, 5, 130
  quantitative, 3, 104, 112
coronary artery spasm, 2
coronary circulation, 4, 5, 13, 17, 18, 21, 33, 39, 141
coronary flow reserve (CFR), xv, 4, 5, 8, 18, 42, 46, 95, 101, 119, 159, 163
  relative, 119
coronary sinus, 13, 19, 153, 162
coronary sinus thermodilution, 19, 20
coronary venous system, 82
cranial angulation, 103
cross-sectional area, 15, 20, 104
cross-sectional flow velocity, 15
Cu-filter, 57, 59
curve fitting, 47, 54, 78, 105, 167
curve parameters, 57
cyclotron, 21, 22

desaturation, 19
diatrizoate (Urographin ^{R}), 40, 57, 153, 154, 156–158, 163
digital subtraction angiography (DSA), xv, 33, 45, 104, 153
  ECG-triggered, 71
dipyridamole, 66, 74–76, 81, 82, 101, 103, 118
dispersion, 94
dissection, 109
distribution function, 31
D_{max}, 81, 89
Doppler
  pulsed, 15

Doppler catheters, 4, 15, 20, 21
Doppler equation, 14
Doppler principle, 15
Doppler probes, 14, 15, 16, 20, 73, 92
Doppler shift, xv, 86
  maximal, 82
  mean, 76
  phasic, 76
dP/dt
  left vertricular, 156
  peak positive, 154
  ventricular, 156
dP/dt_{max}, xv, 157, 163
  left ventricular, 76, 81, 155, 158, 160, 162
droperidol, 73

electrolyte shifts, 162
electromagnetic flow measurement, 14, 64, 66
electromagnetic flow probe, 15, 16, 82, 153
emergency patients, 138, 143
emergency surgery, 109
ethrane, 73
excentricity, 2
excitation-contraction coupling, 162
exercise testing, 5, 102, 112, 118, 121
exercise time, 112
extracorporal circulation, 145
eyeball assessment
  of the stenosis, 109

F-test, 81, 89
Faraday's law of induction, 14
fentanyl, 73
flow
  absolute, 15, 18, 61
  coronary, 4, 15, 18, 21, 28, 33, 39, 155
  densitometric, 58, 64, 65
  electromagnetic, 59, 65
  laminar, 14
  maximal, 5, 8, 21, 42, 43, 102, 103, 120, 122, 129, 142, 143

mean, 39, 154
myocardial, 4, 5, 13, 17, 18, 33, 105, 117, 129
phasic, 154
pulsatile, 39
relative, 15
resting, 4, 5, 8, 95, 101, 102, 119, 142, 144
resting, after PTCA, 120
transmural distribution, 22
turbulent, 14
volumetric, 15, 18, 61, 82
flow model, 48, 55, 62
hydrodynamic, 54
flow velocity, 15, 20
mean, 74
phasic, 74
fluid dynamics, 2
focus size, 2
frequency response, 16, 18
frequency shift, 15
functional improvement, 102, 122, 142, 143, 147
functional success, 116

gamma camera, 17
gamma counter, 17
gamma function, 47, 57, 59, 105, 132, 137, 167, 168, 169, 170
gamma-emitting isotopes, 17
Ganz, 19
gas clearance methods, 19
Gould, xi, 4, 119
guiding catheter, 103

Hamilton, 28
He, 19
heart rate, 103, 131, 144, 155, 158, 159
heart weight, 18
heparin, 154
Hering, 27
hyperemia, 5, 19, 46, 76, 91, 162
contrast-induced, 72, 152
coronary, 142

maximal, 66, 102, 110, 112, 118, 134
myocardial, 142
reactive, 154
hyperemic response, 40, 42
hyperemic stimulus, 4, 20, 46
hyperosmolality, 152, 162
hypertension, 5
hypoperfusion, 145, 146

image acquisition, 45, 47, 55, 75
X-ray synchronous, 104, 117
image noise, 91
image processing, 75, 108, 130, 131
image quality, 109, 121, 134
imaging variables, 131
indicator, 28–31, 33, 39, 42, 63
inert, 151
instantaneous injection, 29
indicator dilution curve, 29, 30, 32, 45, 53
indicator dilution theory, 27, 28, 33, 39, 40, 47, 53, 71, 95, 141, 143
indocyanine green, 28
injection rate, 65, 75
injection signal, 132
injection site
of the indicator, 42
inotropic state. 152, 161, 162, 164
input signal, 92
iodine, 44, 54
iodine concentration, 152
iodine content, 153
iohexol, 154, 156–158, 163
iohexol-140 (Omnipaque 140^R), 40, 55, 57, 75, 152, 153, 161, 164
Iohexol-350, 104, 130

Judkins catheter, 73, 103, 154, 155

labelling, 17
Lambert-Beer's law, 44, 54, 57–59, 63
Langendorff, 13
least square regression method, 58, 155
left anterior descending artery, xv, 104, 113, 115

diagonal branch, 122
intermediate branch, 122
left anterior oblique, xv
left circumflex artery, xv, 40, 73, 104, 113, 115
  obtuse marginal branch, 73
  posterolateral branch, 122
left coronary artery, xv, 73, 155
left ventricular hypertrophy, 8, 19, 95, 119, 144
linear discriminant analysis, 108
linear model, 81
linear regression, 108, 132
lipid lowering therapy, 18, 42, 119, 122, 147
lognormal fit, 59, 62, 169, 170
lognormal function, 47, 57, 167

magnetic resonance imaging, 22
mammarian artery, 146
manual correction, 170
Marquardt method, 78, 105, 168
mask, 45, 76
  pressure corrected (MFRc), xv, 108, 113, 115
maximal flow ratio (MFR), xv, 101, 105, 109, 112, 116, 119, 121
mean circulation time, *see* mean transit time
mean transit time (T_{mn}), xvi, 8, 19, 31–33, 42, 43, 45–48, 53, 59, 65, 66, 71, 72, 91, 101, 102, 105, 110, 112, 113, 115, 129, 131, 137, 142, 143, 162, 169
  normal arteries, 117, 120
membrane transport, 162
microspheres, 15–17
Millar microtip catheter, 73, 154
motion artifacts, 45
multivessel disease, 121, 144
myocardial depression, 162
myocardial extracellular fluid, 162
myocardial infarction, 8, 145

myocardial perfusion, 4, 13, 19, 32, 34, 39, 73, 162
  disturbance of, 147
  maximal, 101, 113, 138
myocardium
  hibernating, 145
  stunned, 145

Na^+/Ca^{++} ratio, 162
nicomorphine, 73
nitroglycerin, 21
no-reflow phenomenon, 145
norcuron, 76
normal arteries, 117
nose clamp, 47, 102

occlusion, 75, 76, 154, 159
  of the LCx artery, 78
osmolality, 153
over-the-wire balloon, 103
overestimation, 2, 20, 65
overprojection, 63, 78, 105, 121
oxygen, 141
oxygen demand, 152

pacing electrodes, 73, 153
panning, 45
papaverine, 66, 75, 81, 91, 104, 118, 130
papillary muscle
  posteromedian, 104, 132
parametric images, 91
pentobarbital, 73
perfusion-contraction coupling, 145
perspex, 55
positron camera, 21
positron emission tomography (PET), xvi, 4, 21
positron emitting isotopes, 21
posterior septum, 104
potassium ferrocyanide, 27
power injector, 55, 75, 104, 130
pressure, xv
  aortic (AoP), xv, 74, 76, 81, 163
  arterial, 3, 103, 105, 109, 134

intravascular, 14
left ventricular (LVP), xv, 76, 81, 154, 155, 158, 159, 162
venous, 2, 3
ventricular systolic, 156
pressure correction, 135, 138
pressure gradient
transstenotic, 2, 103, 108–110, 112, 116, 118, 119
propranolol, 74
Prussian blue reaction, 27
PTCA, 5, 8, 18, 42, 95, 101, 103, 116, 122, 142, 143
elective, 102
pulse width, 75, 104

radiation spectrum, 57
radioactivity, 18
re-PTCA, 109
recirculation, 39
red blood cells
aggregation, 162
sludging, 162
region of interest (ROI), xvi, 33, 39, 42, 43, 45, 76, 167
background, 78, 82, 105, 132, 167
myocardial, 78, 82, 104, 132
processing of, 108
relative difference, 132, 135
relative error (Er), xv, 57, 59, 78, 82, 105, 109, 132, 168, 169
reproducibility, 59, 82, 108, 109, 118, 129, 169
image acquisition of, 129
image processing of, 129
resistance, 2, 4, 27
arteriolar, 42
capillary, 42
peripheral, 43
restenosis, 118, 119
right coronary artery, 113, 115
Robb, 33
roller pump, 55
runoff, 2

Rutishauser, 21, 28, 33, 71, 141

saline, 28
SAS-software package, 80
saturation, 19
serial lesions, 122
shaping factors, 167
Siemens Bicor, 56, 75, 103, 131
Siemens Digitron-3, 56, 75, 103, 131
single vessel disease, 102, 117, 118, 121, 144
sinus rhythm, 102
snare occluder, 153
sodium content, 153, 162
spectrophotometer, 28
spectroscopy, 17
steady state flow, 53
Stewart, 27
stimulation catheter, 103, 109
subendocardial perfusion, 22
substrate, 141
Swan, 28

temporal resolution, 65
thallium scintigraphy, 102, 103, 109, 121
Thebesian veins, 13
thermistor, 19
thermodilution principle, 19, 28
time constant, 19
time density curve (TDC), xvi, 33, 44, 45, 47, 57, 61, 64, 71, 78, 82, 105, 109, 130, 132, 142, 162
time of maximal contrast intensity (T_{max}), xvi, 46, 58
time of maximal inclination, 46
time parameter, 33, 42, 46, 54, 63, 129
definition of, 80
time $t = 0$
definition of, 131, 132
background corrected, 109, 134, 168
timed venous collection, 13, 15
T_{max}, 66
T_{mn}, 66

transstenotic pressure gradient, 2, 103,
      108–110, 112, 116, 118, 119
trigger unit, 73
triggering, 45, 47, 75, 130
  X-ray synchronous, 47

ultrafast computed tomography, 22
Urographin-370, 40, 57, 153

Van der Werf, 28, 47
variability
  inter-observer, 1, 3, 129
  intra-observer, 1, 3, 129
vascular bed
  myocardial, 2
vascular compartment
  of the heart, 94
vascular volume, 30, 31, 33, 42–44, 46,
      48, 53, 54, 58, 64, 65, 72, 76, 81,
      94, 101, 141, 142, 162
  maximal, 91
vasodilation, 4, 42
  maximal, 75, 95, 103, 104, 105, 118,
      119, 130, 138
verapamil, 153–155, 157–161, 163
videochain, 44
videoclock, 76
videodensitometry, 8, 21, 33, 34, 39, 42,
      47, 48, 72, 129, 137
videopulse, 47
viscosity, 153
Vogel, 43, 46, 72

wash-out phase, 45, 53
Wheatstone bridge, 27
Wilcoxon test, 89
Wood, 33

X-ray generator, 47, 76, 104

zero
  electrical, 154
  occlusive, 154
zero density level, 55
zero flow, 14, 154

Ziedzes des Plantes, 151
Zierler, 28

Developments in Cardiovascular Medicine

1. Ch.T. Lancée (ed.): *Echocardiology.* 1979   ISBN 90-247-2209-8
2. J. Baan, A.C. Arntzenius and E.L. Yellin (eds.): *Cardiac Dynamics.* 1980
     ISBN 90-247-2212-8
3. H.J.Th. Thalen and C.C. Meere (eds.): *Fundamentals of Cardiac Pacing.* 1979
     ISBN 90-247-2245-4
4. H.E. Kulbertus and H.J.J. Wellens (eds.): *Sudden Death.* 1980   ISBN 90-247-2290-X
5. L.S. Dreifus and A.N. Brest (eds.): *Clinical Applications of Cardiovascular Drugs.*
1980   ISBN 90-247-2295-0
6. M.P. Spencer and J.M. Reid: *Cerebrovascular Evaluation with Doppler Ultrasound.*
With contributions by E.C. Brockenbrough, R.S. Reneman, G.I. Thomas and D.L.
Davis. 1981   ISBN 90-247-2384-1
7. D.P. Zipes, J.C. Bailey and V. Elharrar (eds.): *The Slow Inward Current and Cardiac
Arrhythmias.* 1980   ISBN 90-247-2380-9
8. H. Kesteloot and J.V. Joossens (eds.): *Epidemiology of Arterial Blood Pressure.* 1980
     ISBN 90-247-2386-8
9. F.J.Th. Wackers (ed.): *Thallium-201 and Technetium-99m-Pyrophosphate. Myocardial Imaging in the Coronary Care Unit.* 1980   ISBN 90-247-2396-5
10. A. Maseri, C. Marchesi, S. Chierchia and M.G. Trivella (eds.): *Coronary Care Units.*
Proceedings of a European Seminar, held in Pisa, Italy (1978). 1981
     ISBN 90-247-2456-2
11. J. Morganroth, E.N. Moore, L.S. Dreifus and E.L. Michelson (eds.): *The Evaluation of
New Antiarrhythmic Drugs.* Proceedings of the First Symposium on New Drugs and
Devices, held in Philadelphia, Pa., U.S.A. (1980). 1981   ISBN 90-247-2474-0
12. P. Alboni: *Intraventricular Conduction Disturbances.* 1981   ISBN 90-247-2483-X
13. H. Rijsterborgh (ed.): *Echocardiology.* 1981   ISBN 90-247-2491-0
14. G.S. Wagner (ed.): *Myocardial Infarction.* Measurement and Intervention. 1982
     ISBN 90-247-2513-5
15. R.S. Meltzer and J. Roelandt (eds.): *Contrast Echocardiography.* 1982
     ISBN 90-247-2531-3
16. A. Amery, R. Fagard, P. Lijnen and J. Staessen (eds.): *Hypertensive Cardiovascular
Disease.* Pathophysiology and Treatment. 1982   IBSN 90-247-2534-8
17. L.N. Bouman and H.J. Jongsma (eds.): *Cardiac Rate and Rhythm.* Physiological,
Morphological and Developmental Aspects. 1982   ISBN 90-247-2626-3
18. J. Morganroth and E.N. Moore (eds.): *The Evaluation of Beta Blocker and Calcium
Antagonist Drugs.* Proceedings of the 2nd Symposium on New Drugs and Devices,
held in Philadelphia, Pa., U.S.A. (1981). 1982   ISBN 90-247-2642-5
19. M.B. Rosenbaum and M.V. Elizari (eds.): *Frontiers of Cardiac Electrophysiology.*
1983   ISBN 90-247-2663-8
20. J. Roelandt and P.G. Hugenholtz (eds.): *Long-term Ambulatory Electrocardiography.*
1982   ISBN 90-247-2664-6
21. A.A.J. Adgey (ed.): *Acute Phase of Ischemic Heart Disease and Myocardial
Infarction.* 1982   ISBN 90-247-2675-1
22. P. Hanrath, W. Bleifeld and J. Souquet (eds.): *Cardiovascular Diagnosis by
Ultrasound.* Transesophageal, Computerized, Contrast, Doppler Echocardiography.
1982   ISBN 90-247-2692-1

Developments in Cardiovascular Medicine

23. J. Roelandt (ed.): *The Practice of M-Mode and Two-dimensional Echocardiography.*
1983   ISBN 90-247-2745-6
24. J. Meyer, P. Schweizer and R. Erbel (eds.): *Advances in Noninvasive Cardiology.*
Ultrasound, Computed Tomography, Radioisotopes, Digital Angiography. 1983
ISBN 0-89838-576-8
25. J. Morganroth and E.N. Moore (eds.): *Sudden Cardiac Death and Congestive Heart
Failure.* Diagnosis and Treatment. Proceedings of the 3rd Symposium on New Drugs
and Devices, held in Philadelphia, Pa., U.S.A. (1982). 1983   ISBN 0-89838-580-6
26. H.M. Perry Jr. (ed.): *Lifelong Management of Hypertension.* 1983
ISBN 0-89838-582-2
27. E.A. Jaffe (ed.): *Biology of Endothelial Cells.* 1984   ISBN 0-89838-587-3
28. B. Surawicz, C.P. Reddy and E.N. Prystowsky (eds.): *Tachycardias.* 1984
ISBN 0-89838-588-1
29. M.P. Spencer (ed.): *Cardiac Doppler Diagnosis.* Proceedings of a Symposium, held in
Clearwater, Fla., U.S.A. (1983). 1983   ISBN 0-89838-591-1
30. H. Villarreal and M.P. Sambhi (eds.): *Topics in Pathophysiology of Hypertension.*
1984   ISBN 0-89838-595-4
31. F.H. Messerli (ed.): *Cardiovascular Disease in the Elderly.* 1984
Revised edition, 1988: see below under Volume 76
32. M.L. Simoons and J.H.C. Reiber (eds.): *Nuclear Imaging in Clinical Cardiology.*
1984   ISBN 0-89838-599-7
33. H.E.D.J. ter Keurs and J.J. Schipperheyn (eds.): *Cardiac Left Ventricular Hypertrophy.* 1983   ISBN 0-89838-612-8
34. N. Sperelakis (ed.): *Physiology and Pathology of the Heart.* 1984
Revised edition, 1988: see below under Volume 90
35. F.H. Messerli (ed.): *Kidney in Essential Hypertension.* Proceedings of a Course, held
in New Orleans, La., U.S.A. (1983). 1984   ISBN 0-89838-616-0
36. M.P. Sambhi (ed.): *Fundamental Fault in Hypertension.* 1984   ISBN 0-89838-638-1
37. C. Marchesi (ed.): *Ambulatory Monitoring.* Cardiovascular System and Allied
Applications. Proceedings of a Workshop, held in Pisa, Italy (1983). 1984
ISBN 0-89838-642-X
38. W. Kupper, R.N. MacAlpin and W. Bleifeld (eds.): *Coronary Tone in Ischemic Heart
Disease.* 1984   ISBN 0-89838-646-2
39. N. Sperelakis and J.B. Caulfield (eds.): *Calcium Antagonists.* Mechanism of Action
on Cardiac Muscle and Vascular Smooth Muscle. Proceedings of the 5th Annual
Meeting of the American Section of the I.S.H.R., held in Hilton Head, S.C., U.S.A.
(1983). 1984   ISBN 0-89838-655-1
40. Th. Godfraind, A.G. Herman and D. Wellens (eds.): *Calcium Entry Blockers in
Cardiovascular and Cerebral Dysfunctions.* 1984   ISBN 0-89838-658-6
41. J. Morganroth and E.N. Moore (eds.): *Interventions in the Acute Phase of Myocardial
Infarction.* Proceedings of the 4th Symposium on New Drugs and Devices, held in
Philadelphia, Pa., U.S.A. (1983). 1984   ISBN 0-89838-659-4
42. F.L. Abel and W.H. Newman (eds.): *Functional Aspects of the Normal, Hyper-
trophied and Failing Heart.* Proceedings of the 5th Annual Meeting of the American
Section of the I.S.H.R., held in Hilton Head, S.C., U.S.A. (1983). 1984
ISBN 0-89838-665-9

Developments in Cardiovascular Medicine

43. S. Sideman and R. Beyar (eds.): [3-D] *Simulation and Imaging of the Cardiac System.* State of the Heart. Proceedings of the International Henry Goldberg Workshop, held in Haifa, Israel (1984). 1985   ISBN 0-89838-687-X

44. E. van der Wall and K.I. Lie (eds.): *Recent Views on Hypertrophic Cardiomyopathy.* Proceedings of a Symposium, held in Groningen, The Netherlands (1984). 1985
                                                                                     ISBN 0-89838-694-2

45. R.E. Beamish, P.K. Singal and N.S. Dhalla (eds.), *Stress and Heart Disease.* Proceedings of a International Symposium, held in Winnipeg, Canada, 1984 (Vol. 1). 1985   ISBN 0-89838-709-4

46. R.E. Beamish, V. Panagia and N.S. Dhalla (eds.): *Pathogenesis of Stress-induced Heart Disease.* Proceedings of a International Symposium, held in Winnipeg, Canada, 1984 (Vol. 2). 1985   ISBN 0-89838-710-8

47. J. Morganroth and E.N. Moore (eds.): *Cardiac Arrhythmias.* New Therapeutic Drugs and Devices. Proceedings of the 5th Symposium on New Drugs and Devices, held in Philadelphia, Pa., U.S.A. (1984). 1985   ISBN 0-89838-716-7

48. P. Mathes (ed.): *Secondary Prevention in Coronary Artery Disease and Myocardial Infarction.* 1985   ISBN 0-89838-736-1

49. H.L. Stone and W.B. Weglicki (eds.): *Pathobiology of Cardiovascular Injury.* Proceedings of the 6th Annual Meeting of the American Section of the I.S.H.R., held in Oklahoma City, Okla., U.S.A. (1984). 1985   ISBN 0-89838-743-4

50. J. Meyer, R. Erbel and H.J. Rupprecht (eds.): *Improvement of Myocardial Perfusion.* Thrombolysis, Angioplasty, Bypass Surgery. Proceedings of a Symposium, held in Mainz, F.R.G. (1984). 1985   ISBN 0-89838-748-5

51. J.H.C. Reiber, P.W. Serruys and C.J. Slager (eds.): *Quantitative Coronary and Left Ventricular Cineangiography.* Methodology and Clinical Applications. 1986
                                                                                     ISBN 0-89838-760-4

52. R.H. Fagard and I.E. Bekaert (eds.): *Sports Cardiology.* Exercise in Health and Cardiovascular Disease. Proceedings from an International Conference, held in Knokke, Belgium (1985). 1986   ISBN 0-89838-782-5

53. J.H.C. Reiber and P.W. Serruys (eds.): *State of the Art in Quantitative Cornary Arteriography.* 1986   ISBN 0-89838-804-X

54. J. Roelandt (ed.): *Color Doppler Flow Imaging and Other Advances in Doppler Echocardiography.* 1986   ISBN 0-89838-806-6

55. E.E. van der Wall (ed.): *Noninvasive Imaging of Cardiac Metabolism.* Single Photon Scintigraphy, Positron Emission Tomography and Nuclear Magnetic Resonance. 1987
                                                                                     ISBN 0-89838-812-0

56. J. Liebman, R. Plonsey and Y. Rudy (eds.): *Pediatric and Fundamental Electrocardiography.* 1987   ISBN 0-89838-815-5

57. H.H. Hilger, V. Hombach and W.J. Rashkind (eds.), *Invasive Cardiovascular Therapy.* Proceedings of an International Symposium, held in Cologne, F.R.G. (1985). 1987   ISBN 0-89838-818-X

58. P.W. Serruys and G.T. Meester (eds.): *Coronary Angioplasty.* A Controlled Model for Ischemia. 1986   ISBN 0-89838-819-8

59. J.E. Tooke and L.H. Smaje (eds.): *Clinical Investigation of the Microcirculation.* Proceedings of an International Meeting, held in London, U.K. (1985). 1987
                                                                                     ISBN 0-89838-833-3

Developments in Cardiovascular Medicine

60. R.Th. van Dam and A. van Oosterom (eds.): *Electrocardiographic Body Surface Mapping*. Proceedings of the 3rd International Symposium on B.S.M., held in Nijmegen, The Netherlands (1985). 1986   ISBN 0-89838-834-1

61. M.P. Spencer (ed.): *Ultrasonic Diagnosis of Cerebrovascular Disease*. Doppler Techniques and Pulse Echo Imaging. 1987   ISBN 0-89838-836-8

62. M.J. Legato (ed.): *The Stressed Heart*. 1987   ISBN 0-89838-849-X

63. M.E. Safar (ed.): *Arterial and Venous Systems in Essential Hypertension*. With Assistance of G.M. London, A.Ch. Simon and Y.A. Weiss. 1987

     ISBN 0-89838-857-0

64. J. Roelandt (ed.): *Digital Techniques in Echocardiography*. 1987

     ISBN 0-89838-861-9

65. N.S. Dhalla, P.K. Singal and R.E. Beamish (eds.): *Pathology of Heart Disease*. Proceedings of the 8th Annual Meeting of the American Section of the I.S.H.R., held in Winnipeg, Canada, 1986 (Vol. 1). 1987   ISBN 0-89838-864-3

66. N.S. Dhalla, G.N. Pierce and R.E. Beamish (eds.): *Heart Function and Metabolism*. Proceedings of the 8th Annual Meeting of the American Section of the I.S.H.R., held in Winnipeg, Canada, 1986 (Vol. 2). 1987   ISBN 0-89838-865-1

67. N.S. Dhalla, I.R. Innes and R.E. Beamish (eds.): *Myocardial Ischemia*. Proceedings of a Satellite Symposium of the 30th International Physiological Congress, held in Winnipeg, Canada (1986). 1987   ISBN 0-89838-866-X

68. R.E. Beamish, V. Panagia and N.S. Dhalla (eds.): *Pharmacological Aspects of Heart Disease*. Proceedings of an International Symposium, held in Winnipeg, Canada (1986). 1987   ISBN 0-89838-867-8

69. H.E.D.J. ter Keurs and J.V. Tyberg (eds.): *Mechanics of the Circulation*. Proceedings of a Satellite Symposium of the 30th International Physiological Congress, held in Banff, Alberta, Canada (1986). 1987   ISBN 0-89838-870-8

70. S. Sideman and R. Beyar (eds.): *Activation, Metabolism and Perfusion of the Heart*. Simulation and Experimental Models. Proceedings of the 3rd Henry Goldberg Workshop, held in Piscataway, N.J., U.S.A. (1986). 1987   ISBN 0-89838-871-6

71. E. Aliot and R. Lazzara (eds.): *Ventricular Tachycardias*. From Mechanism to Therapy. 1987   ISBN 0-89838-881-3

72. A. Schneeweiss and G. Schettler: *Cardiovascular Drug Therapoy in the Elderly*. 1988

     ISBN 0-89838-883-X

73. J.V. Chapman and A. Sgalambro (eds.): *Basic Concepts in Doppler Echocardiography*. Methods of Clinical Applications based on a Multi-modality Doppler Approach. 1987   ISBN 0-89838-888-0

74. S. Chien, J. Dormandy, E. Ernst and A. Matrai (eds.): *Clinical Hemorheology*. Applications in Cardiovascular and Hematological Disease, Diabetes, Surgery and Gynecology. 1987   ISBN 0-89838-807-4

75. J. Morganroth and E.N. Moore (eds.): *Congestive Heart Failure*. Proceedings of the 7th Annual Symposium on New Drugs and Devices, held in Philadelphia, Pa., U.S.A. (1986). 1987   ISBN 0-89838-955-0

76. F.H. Messerli (ed.): *Cardiovascular Disease in the Elderly*. 2nd ed. 1988

     ISBN 0-89838-962-3

77. P.H. Heintzen and J.H. Bürsch (eds.): *Progress in Digital Angiocardiography*. 1988

     ISBN 0-89838-965-8

Developments in Cardiovascular Medicine

78. M.M. Scheinman (ed.): *Catheter Ablation of Cardiac Arrhythmias.* Basic Bioelectrical Effects and Clinical Indications. 1988   ISBN 0-89838-967-4
79. J.A.E. Spaan, A.V.G. Bruschke and A.C. Gittenberger-De Groot (eds.): *Coronary Circulation.* From Basic Mechanisms to Clinical Implications. 1987
ISBN 0-89838-978-X
80. C. Visser, G. Kan and R.S. Meltzer (eds.): *Echocardiography in Coronary Artery Disease.* 1988   ISBN 0-89838-979-8
81. A. Bayés de Luna, A. Betriu and G. Permanyer (eds.): *Therapeutics in Cardiology.* 1988   ISBN 0-89838-981-X
82. D.M. Mirvis (ed.): *Body Surface Electrocardiographic Mapping.* 1988
ISBN 0-89838-983-6
83. M.A. Konstam and J.M. Isner (eds.): *The Right Ventricle.* 1988   ISBN 0-89838-987-9
84. C.T. Kappagoda and P.V. Greenwood (eds.): *Long-term Management of Patients after Myocardial Infarction.* 1988   ISBN 0-89838-352-8
85. W.H. Gaasch and H.J. Levine (eds.): *Chronic Aortic Regurgitation.* 1988
ISBN 0-89838-364-1
86. P.K. Singal (ed.): *Oxygen Radicals in the Pathophysiology of Heart Disease.* 1988
ISBN 0-89838-375-7
87. J.H.C. Reiber and P.W. Serruys (eds.): *New Developments in Quantitative Coronary Arteriography.* 1988   ISBN 0-89838-377-3
88. J. Morganroth and E.N. Moore (eds.): *Silent Myocardial Ischemia.* Proceedings of the 8th Annual Symposium on New Drugs and Devices (1987). 1988
ISBN 0-89838-380-3
89. H.E.D.J. ter Keurs and M.I.M. Noble (eds.): *Starling's Law of the Heart Revisted.* 1988   ISBN 0-89838-382-X
90. N. Sperelakis (ed.): *Physiology and Pathophysiology of the Heart.* (Rev. ed.) 1988
ISBN 0-89838-388-9
91. J.W. de Jong (ed.): *Myocardial Energy Metabolism.* 1988   ISBN 0-89838-394-3
92. V. Hombach, H.H. Hilger and H.L. Kennedy (eds.): *Electrocardiography and Cardiac Drug Therapy.* Proceedings of an International Symposium, held in Cologne, F.R.G. (1987). 1988   ISBN 0-89838-395-1
93. H. Iwata, J.B. Lombardini and T. Segawa (eds.): *Taurine and the Heart.* 1988
ISBN 0-89838-396-X
94. M.R. Rosen and Y. Palti (eds.): *Lethal Arrhythmias Resulting from Myocardial Ischemia and Infarction.* Proceedings of the 2nd Rappaport Symposium, held in Haifa, Israel (1988). 1988   ISBN 0-89838-401-X
95. M. Iwase and I. Sotobata: *Clinical Echocardiography.* With a Foreword by M.P. Spencer. 1989   ISBN 0-7923-0004-1
96. I. Cikes (ed.): *Echocardiography in Cardiac Interventions.* 1989
ISBN 0-7923-0088-2
97. E. Rapaport (ed.): *Early Interventions in Acute Myocardial Infarction.* 1989
ISBN 0-7923-0175-7
98. M.E. Safar and F. Fouad-Tarazi (eds.): *The Heart in Hypertension.* A Tribute to Robert C. Tarazi (1925-1986). 1989   ISBN 0-7923-0197-8
99. S. Meerbaum and R. Meltzer (eds.): *Myocardial Contrast Two-dimensional Echocardiography.* 1989   ISBN 0-7923-0205-2

Developments in Cardiovascular Medicine

100. J. Morganroth and E.N. Moore (eds.): *Risk/Benefit Analysis for the Use and Approval of Thrombolytic, Antiarrhythmic, and Hypolipidemic Agents*. Proceedings of the 9th Annual Symposium on New Drugs and Devices (1988). 1989   ISBN 0-7923-0294-X

101. P.W. Serruys, R. Simon and K.J. Beatt (eds.): *PTCA - An Investigational Tool and a Non-operative Treatment of Acute Ischemia*. 1990   ISBN 0-7923-0346-6

102. I.S. Anand, P.I. Wahi and N.S. Dhalla (eds.): *Pathophysiology and Pharmacology of Heart Disease*. 1989   ISBN 0-7923-0367-9

103. G.S. Abela (ed.): *Lasers in Cardiovascular Medicine and Surgery*. Fundamentals and Technique. 1990   ISBN 0-7923-0440-3

104. H.M. Piper (ed.): *Pathophysiology of Severe Ischemic Myocardial Injury*. 1990
ISBN 0-7923-0459-4

105. S.M. Teague (ed.): *Stress Doppler Echocardiography*. 1990   ISBN 0-7923-0499-3

106. P.R. Saxena, D.I. Wallis, W. Wouters and P. Bevan (eds.): *Cardiovascular Pharmacology of 5-Hydroxytryptamine*. Prospective Therapeutic Applications. 1990
ISBN 0-7923-0502-7

107. A.P. Shepherd and P.A. Öberg (eds.): *Laser-Doppler Blood Flowmetry*. 1990
ISBN 0-7923-0508-6

108. J. Soler-Soler, G. Permanyer-Miralda and J. Sagristà-Sauleda (eds.): *Pericardial Disease*. New Insights and Old Dilemmas. Preface by Ralph Shabetai. 1990
ISBN 0-7923-0510-8

109. J.P.M. Hamer: *Practical Echocardiography in the Adult*. With Doppler and Color-Doppler Flow Imaging. 1990   ISBN 0-7923-0670-8

110. A. Bayés de Luna, P. Brugada, J. Cosin Aguilar and F. Navarro Lopez (eds.): *Sudden Cardiac Death*. 1991   ISBN 0-7923-0716-X

111. E. Andries and R. Stroobandt (eds.): *Hemodynamics in Daily Practice*. 1991
ISBN 0-7923-0725-9

112. J. Morganroth and E.N. Moore (eds.): *Use and Approval of Antihypertensive Agents and Surrogate Endpoints for the Approval of Drugs affecting Antiarrhythmic Heart Failure and Hypolipidemia*. Proceedings of the 10th Annual Symposium on New Drugs and Devices (1989). 1990   ISBN 0-7923-0756-9

113. S. Iliceto, P. Rizzon and J.R.T.C. Roelandt (eds.): *Ultrasound in Coronary Artery Disease*. Present Role and Future Perspectives. 1990   ISBN 0-7923-0784-4

114. J.V. Chapman and G.R. Sutherland (eds.): *The Noninvasive Evaluation of Hemodynamics in Congenital Heart Disease*. Doppler Ultrasound Applications in the Adult and Pediatric Patient with Congenital Heart Disease. 1990
ISBN 0-7923-0836-0

115. G.T. Meester and F. Pinciroli (eds.): *Databases for Cardiology*. 1991
ISBN 0-7923-0886-7

116. B. Korecky and N.S. Dhalla (eds.): *Subcellular Basis of Contractile Failure*. 1990
ISBN 0-7923-0890-5

117. J.H.C. Reiber and P.W. Serruys (eds.): *Quantitative Coronary Arteriography*. 1991
ISBN 0-7923-0913-8

118. E. van der Wall and A. de Roos (eds.): *Magnetic Resonance Imaging in Coronary Artery Disease*. 1991   ISBN 0-7923-0940-5

119. V. Hombach, M. Kochs and A.J. Camm (eds.): *Interventional Techniques in Cardiovascular Medicine*. 1991   ISBN 0-7923-0956-1

Developments in Cardiovascular Medicine

120. R. Vos: *Drugs Looking for Diseases*. Innovative Drug Research and the Development of the Beta Blockers and the Calcium Antagonists. 1991   ISBN 0-7923-0968-5
121. S. Sideman, R. Beyar and A. G. Kleber (eds.): *Cardiac Electrophysiology, Circulation, and Transport*. Proceedings of the 7th Henry Goldberg Workshop (Berne, Switzerland, 1990). 1991   ISBN 0-7923-1145-0
122. D.M. Bers: *Excitation-Contraction Coupling and Cardiac Contractile Force*. 1991
          ISBN 0-7923-1186-8
123. A.-M. Salmasi and A.N. Nicolaides (eds.): *Occult Atherosclerotic Disease*. Diagnosis, Assessment and Management. 1991   ISBN 0-7923-1188-4
124. J.A.E. Spaan: *Coronary Blood Flow*. Mechanics, Distribution, and Control. 1991
          ISBN 0-7923-1210-4
125. R.W. Stout (ed.): *Diabetes and Atherosclerosis*. 1991   ISBN 0-7923-1310-0
126. A.G. Herman (ed.): *Antithrombotics*. Pathophysiological Rationale for Pharmacological Interventions. 1991   ISBN 0-7923-1413-1
127. N.H.J. Pijls: *Maximal Myocardial Perfusion as a Measure of the Functional Significance of Coronary Artery Disease*. 1991   ISBN 0-7923-1430-1

Previous volumes are still available

KLUWER ACADEMIC PUBLISHERS – DORDRECHT / BOSTON / LONDON